Feederism

DOI: 10.1057/9781137470461.0001

Other Palgrave Pivot titles

Brendan Howe: **Democratic Governance in Northeast Asia: A Human-Centred Approach to Evaluating Democracy**

Evie Kendal: **Equal Opportunity and the Case for State Sponsored Ectogenesis**

Joseph Watras: **Philosophies of Environmental Education and Democracy: Harris, Dewey, and Bateson on Human Freedoms in Nature**

Christos Kourtelis: **The Political Economy of Euro-Mediterranean Relations: European Neighbourhood Policy in North Africa**

Liz Montegary and Melissa Autumn White (*editors*): **Mobile Desires: The Politics and Erotics of Mobility Justice**

Anna Larsson and Sanja Magdalenić: **Sociology in Sweden: A History**

Philip Whitehead: **Reconceptualising the Moral Economy of Criminal Justice: A New Perspective**

Robert Kerr: **How Postmodernism Explains Football and Football Explains Postmodernism: The Billy Clyde Conundrum**

Ilan Bijaoui: **The Open Incubator Model: Entrepreneurship, Open Innovation, and Economic Development in the Periphery**

Pilar Melero: **Mythological Constructs of Mexican Femininity**

Rafael Kandiyoti: **Powering Europe: Russia, Ukraine, and the Energy Squeeze**

Cristina Sánchez-Conejero: **Sex and Ethics in Spanish Cinema**

Matthew Gritter: **The Policy and Politics of Food Stamps and SNAP**

Bridget Kevane: **The Dynamics of Jewish Latino Relationships: Hope and Caution**

Nataly Z. Chesky, Mark R. Wolfmeyer: **Philosophy of STEM Education: A Critical Investigation**

Seung Ho Park, Gerardo R. Ungson, and Andrew Cosgrove: **Scaling the Tail: Managing Profitable Growth in Emerging Markets**

David Michalski: **The Dialectic of Taste: On the Rise and Fall of Tuscanization and other Crises in the Aesthetic Economy**

Adam Okulicz-Kozaryn: **Happiness and Place: Why Life is Better Outside of the City**

Palash Kamruzzaman: **Dollarisation of Poverty: Rethinking Poverty Beyond 2015**

John A. Mathews, Hao Tan: **China's Renewable Energy Revolution**

DOI: 10.1057/9781137470461.0001

palgrave▸pivot

Feederism: Eating, Weight Gain, and Sexual Pleasure

Kathy Charles

Lecturer, Edinburgh Napier University, UK

and

Michael Palkowski

Edinburgh Napier University, UK

palgrave macmillan

DOI: 10.1057/9781137470461.0001

First published 2015 by
PALGRAVE MACMILLAN

Palgrave Macmillan in the UK is an imprint of Macmillan Publishers Limited, registered in England, company number 785998, of Houndmills, Basingstoke, Hampshire RG21 6XS.

Palgrave Macmillan in the US is a division of St Martin's Press LLC, 175 Fifth Avenue, New York, NY 10010.

Palgrave Macmillan is the global academic imprint of the above companies and has companies and representatives throughout the world.

Palgrave® and Macmillan® are registered trademarks in the United States, the United Kingdom, Europe and other countries.

ISBN: 978–1–137–47047–8 EPUB
ISBN: 978–1–137–47046–1 PDF
ISBN: 978–1–137–47045–4 Hardback

A catalogue record for this book is available from the British Library.

A catalog record for this book is available from the Library of Congress.

www.palgrave.com/pivot

DOI: 10.1057/9781137470461

Contents

Personal Acknowledgements vi

Formal Acknowledgements vii

Introduction viii

1 Feederism in Context: Mainstream Depictions, Psychology, and Sociology 1

2 Personal Stories and Feederism Fiction 40

3 Future Directions for Feederism 89

Index 100

Personal Acknowledgements

We would like to thank all the participants in this research who trusted us with their personal stories. We would also like to thank the many people who volunteered but were not able to take part due to our deadlines.

DOI: 10.1057/9781137470461.0002

Formal Acknowledgements

Thank you to Gabriela for the cover of the first edition of *HORNGRY Magazine*. Image courtesy of Gabriela TenderLovingCares, creator and editor of *HORNGRY Magazine*.

Introduction

This text is the most comprehensive published discussion of feederism currently available. The first chapter offers an analysis of what is currently known about feederism and how it has been studied. The authors present the mainstream depictions available such as documentaries, films, websites, and journalism. They then analyse the psychological research carried out to date, which mainly focuses on feederism as a form of masochism or other paraphilia. Psychological ideas concerning addiction and evolutionary mechanisms are also discussed, in an effort to give the fullest picture of how psychological understanding has contributed to knowledge in this area. The second half of the chapter is dedicated to the work of sociologists and spans research encompassing fat studies, stigmatized identities, and historical perspectives on sexuality. Considerable space is also given to a critical appraisal of the feminist perspective taken by much of the previous research. The first chapter concludes by highlighting some of the methodological limitations of previous research into feederism.

The second chapter presents new data gathered from the feederism community. A thematic analysis of 23 participants is presented in three blocks. Seven participants who took part in an interview by writing their answers are analysed first, followed by ten individuals who answered questions conversationally in real time, and finally six participants in the form of three couples who also answered questions in real time. In addition to this new data, a thematic analysis of five pieces of feederism fiction is also

DOI: 10.1057/9781137470461.0004

presented. This chapter gives authentic commentaries from participants adopting a variety of feederism roles (e.g. feeders, feedees, and mutual gainers), and it also offers the first-ever analysis of couples engaged in feederism practices. The key themes that emerge from these analyses are an early attraction to fat, agency, and fantasy. Childhood fascination with fat is very common, and issues of agency are of considerable importance to this community, as they have often been depicted as coercive and deeply pathological individuals. The importance of fantasy as a place to explore the extremes of feederism is also discussed, as real-life interest in issues such as immobility is very limited. The sociological analysis of five feederism stories supplements the interviews by presenting alternative ways of understanding the lived world and different identities. Feederism fiction allows extreme and "deviant" fantasies and identities to be explored safely.

The final chapter brings together the findings of Chapter 2 to offer a theoretical contribution, an analysis of the practical applications of this work, and suggestions for where feederism research can go next. It is argued that attempting to understand feederism using a psychological framework of pathology is inappropriate. The childhood attraction to fat and lifelong interest and erotic feelings for it into adulthood suggests a form of sexuality more so than a fetish. The desire of psychology to explain feederism as a paraphilia limits research in this area and continues to stigmatize it as a "deviant" sexual practice. The non-coercive nature of feederism, and the potential happiness it can bring to those who practice it, are discussed in a health context and it is suggested that awareness of feederism should be increased among medical professionals. The ways in which obese individuals can remain active and healthy is discussed along with recent research supporting the value of the "Health at Every Size" message in encouraging exercise. Future research into feederism should explore more diverse research methods and populations. There is currently no quantitative research on this subject, and ideas for this are discussed along with suggestions for autoethnographic accounts – particularly from women who have previously been regarded as "victims" of feederism rather than legitimate participants. Cultural and sexual diversity in feederism is also an area for new work. Most research has focussed on North America and Europe and has also centred on heterosexual relationships (despite a considerable quantity of gay feederism activity online). The limitations of the new research are also discussed, with the main focus being participant demographics.

DOI: 10.1057/9781137470461.0004

1

Feederism in Context: Mainstream Depictions, Psychology, and Sociology

Abstract: *This chapter explores mainstream depictions of feederism and erotic weight gain, alongside an analysis of psychological and sociological research in this field. Mainstream portrayals come from documentaries, films, journalism, and websites. Psychological analysis encompasses studies on masochism and other paraphilia, evolutionary mechanisms, and addiction. Sociological work to date has often taken a feminist perspective regarding feederism as part of a patriarchal power dynamic. The feminist perspective is critically appraised alongside studies into stigmatized identities and framing. This chapter also highlights some of the methodological limitations in previous feederism research.*

Charles, Kathy and Michael Palkowski. *Feederism: Eating, Weight Gain, and Sexual Pleasure.* Basingstoke: Palgrave Macmillan, 2015. DOI: 10.1057/9781137470461.0005.

Introduction

This chapter provides a systematic review of the academic literature available on feederism and outlines connections that can be made with other fields of inquiry, such as the sociology of the body, fat studies, the psychology of addiction, and paraphilia. The chapter also describes the online spaces where feederism is talked about as a lifestyle and reflects on the gendered diversity of the community. Attention is paid to providing a historical background to sexuality and considering the issue of fat in other cultures. Feederism is placed within a wider context – out with the individual – by recognizing the macro social and cultural issues surrounding it. It is also considered at the individual level by looking at psychological issues relating to paraphilia and evaluating briefly the literature which links feederism to masochism. The literature discussed here acts as context for the present research and themes that are discussed in detail in Chapter 2. To date there have been no attempts at a comprehensive review of the literature available on feederism, so this chapter addresses that gap by critically discussing and evaluating the main theories and methodological work available.

It is necessary to outline some of the terminology used within the feederism community. The range of terminology associated with feederism varies depending on the perspective, role, and sexuality of the person using it. For the purposes of this book, "feederism" refers to a sexual interest where individuals are sexually aroused by either gaining weight themselves (feedee) or by helping another person to gain weight (feeder). A person may adopt both of these roles simultaneously (mutual gainer) or at different points in their lives and relationships. The word feederism itself is contested, with some individuals preferring feedism. For some, feederism suggests that the feeder is dominant and that the feedee is simply the recipient of another person's wishes, whereas feedism suggests a more equal relationship between the feeder and feedee. The word feeder is also shunned by some who may prefer "encourager" or "feedist" – again reflecting a more consensual situation rather than one where the feeder is dominant. Equally, feedee is sometimes replaced with "gainer" which suggests a more active role on the part of the person gaining weight. Although feederism, feeder, and feedee are all used in this research, this by no means undermines or rejects other terminologies. The considerable range of terminology that is used in indicating sexual preferences for erotic weight gain is indicative of the different

DOI: 10.1057/9781137470461.0005

types of people engaging in feederism. These terms can also overlap into other sexual fetishes such as financial domination (e.g. niche forms of financial domination where feedees have "pay pigs" fund their extravagant calorific meals). It is also helpful to acknowledge that feederism is referred to variously as a fetish, a subculture, a kink, and a sexual preference. While these terms can have very different meanings, they are often used interchangeably by researchers and people in the feederism community. As such, the same terms are used throughout this text.

Mainstream representations of feederism

It is worthwhile to briefly outline the ways in which people involved in feederism network and engage with the ideas and lifestyle of the fetish online. Fantasy Feeder is a website that is commonly used as an entry point for those interested in feederism and is immediately accessible. The site has forums and photographs and the aim of the site is to offer a welcoming space for those engaging in feederism. The site caters to a much larger audience than sites such as *Dimensions Magazine* (*Dimensions* was a print magazine initially and had an early online presence), which has lots of user generated fiction on a whole range of different scenarios and fantasies. Weight stories are a significant part of the community and are a way of exploring and testing out new kinks and identities that might not be possible in real life. *Dimensions* was once considered an entry point into feederism in much the same way that Fantasy Feeder currently is today. Old magazine columns and postings are saved in an online library, which is accessible to everyone. *Dimensions* also has a page called The 900 Club, which is a hall of fame for the world's fattest people. The list features 28 people who have gained extraordinary amounts of weight and provides brief biographical descriptions of them alongside photographs and sources. The website has a variety of interesting pieces of fiction which will be discussed more in depth in Chapter 2.

The blogging site Tumblr has an impressive amount of personal pages with people discussing feederism. These are mostly photographic, but they include a wealth of diary entries, goals and lists. There are also user-generated gif images and videos of people showing their fat. Some of the photographs are essentially soft-core pornography. Many of the photographs feature before and after shots with a smaller-sized stomach growing larger. The Tumblr posts usually reflect a wide range of gendered

DOI: 10.1057/9781137470461.0005

identities and ages, and the diversity of the community is evident. The pages available also feature Photoshopping of popular celebrities to have larger bodies. Many of the themes that are shared are ideas of excess and being gluttonous. Information-sharing and discussion on feederism is extremely active and receives many reposts. This impressive diversity is not reflected in mainstream portrayals of the fetish, and Tumblr has not been discussed in previous feederism research.

Alternative sources exist that focus on other aspects of the community, such as *HORNGRY* (tenderlovingcares, 2015) an online magazine which caters to women who want to be or are feeders to men, and ExtremeFeeding, a site dedicated to more extreme feederism, such as the use of equipment to maximize the amount of food a person can ingest. *HORNGRY* is discussed further in Chapter 2. The website extremefeeding.com (run by "Ruben") contains photographs, blog posts, podcasts, fictional stories, poems, and links, all relating to feederism. People can comment on the website and share their own experiences. This site has been referred to by other researchers in this field (e.g. Prohaska, 2013). One of Ruben's blog posts covers the topics of force-feeding and tube-feeding (ExtremeFeeding, 2012a) in detail. He describes how to insert the tube, how to feed the feedee so that permanent damage is not caused, and how to establish safe words or a system of pointing at traffic light colours to indicate whether the process should stop or continue. Ruben claims to have experienced forced tube-feeding himself and emphasizes the need to have a profoundly trusting relationship between the feeder and feedee (who is sometimes tied down during the feeding). This description is very similar to what one might find regarding more typical sadomasochism practices, such as bondage. Masochism is also evident when Ruben claims, "to call a person that is hot for tube feeding a lard tub, a sack of fat or fat sow, or jiggling sagging fat porker is not offensive or insulting, many people that are into such extreme weight gain love to be called things like this, it underlines what they really are and already know" (ExtremeFeeding, 2012a). There are obvious parallels here with the messages a dominatrix might use when dominating a client.

Ruben identifies himself as male feedee, yet he also writes extensively about the feeder role and feeding a woman to immobility. In his poem "Immobile" he describes the process of eagerly feeing a woman to immobility and how she wants the same thing. As with other extreme material on feederism, the focus on fattening eclipses the focus on food in every

DOI: 10.1057/9781137470461.0005

instance, with Ruben preferring to concentrate on seeing a woman grow "And now you are, a sculpture of fat, something to admire and worship" (ExtremeFeeding, 2012b). The many animal (cow, pig, sow) and inanimate object (tub of lard, lard bucket) references in feederism writing are interesting. The feedee becomes a thing rather than a man or woman with a personality or their own wishes. They are transformed into an object that can be altered by the feeder. The ExtremeFeeding site is full of examples of wanting to attach equipment to a feedee like an animal or to feed them in an industrial environment so the mechanized aspect of feeding can be heightened. The goal of immobility clearly adds to this dehumanizing by taking away the feedee's ability to move or fully express themselves.

Returning to the mainstream representations depicting feederism, television documentaries are a popular medium for showcasing the fetish, and they have had a significant impact on forming attitudes towards the behaviours associated with feederism. These portrayals, often negative, have generated press coverage focusing on the deleterious and damaging effects feederism has on health, with links being made to domestic violence. In 2003 Optomen Television released the documentary "Fat Girls and Feeders" in the UK. Now more than 10 years old, this documentary is still broadcast occasionally and is relatively well-known as a depiction of feederism. It has also been screened widely outside of the UK. The documentary is described by the "Really" channel as "a look at the sub-culture of 'feeders' – men who continue to feed large women to encourage them to gain more weight to the point where the women become immobile and risk their lives. Featuring interviews with both the male feeders and the women they feed" (Really, 2014).

This is an accurate description of the film, which mainly focuses on the relationship between Mark and his wife, Gina. Mark's desire is for Gina to become the world's fattest woman, and he appears to become sexually aroused at her increasing immobility. She eventually reaches more than 800lbs and requires constant care. When Gina eventually begins to lose weight Mark's disappointment seems palpable. The documentary provoked a strong response from many people who wrote damning evaluations of Mark and the implied sinister motivations. A highly comment-yielding blog post by Martin (2010) illustrates this: "feeders prey upon vulnerability and insecurity... their goal is to literally trap someone in their own body and this is a form of kidnapping. It is absolutely Machiavellian..."

DOI: 10.1057/9781137470461.0005

Each time "Fat Girls and Feeders" is screened, it provokes a similar response from a new audience. The portrayal of Mark is difficult to like, and the helplessness of Gina is difficult to watch. Yet while this documentary is well-known, and often referred to in journalistic writing on feederism, to what extent is it an accurate portrayal of the subculture of feederism? In 2008, Donna Simpson declared that she wanted to become the world's fattest woman and set herself a target weight of 1000 lbs. She received global media coverage. The relevance of Simpson is that much of her eating was broadcast online, where men would pay $19 per month to watch and encourage her to eat – including the consumption of a 30,000 calorie Christmas dinner. She also had male partners who are reported to have found her weight gain "sexy" and facilitated her goal. After separating from her partner in 2011, Simpson decided to close down her pay-per-view website and go on a diet. She wrote an announcement on her website suggesting that her time in the feederism subculture was a mistake "I was in a relationship that was based on a fetish that exists only in a fantasy" (Simpson, 2014). This appears to be another highly publicized example of feederism in which a woman became the victim of a man or men who wished to feed her to destruction.

In the discussions that follow online postings about the kind of feederism depicted in the cases of Gina and Donna Simpson, there are typically a range of reactions. There is disgust that a person could become so large, anger and distress at the apparent abusive nature of the relationship, attempts to understand the psychology of the relationship, speculation that the feedee may be mentally ill and/or the feeder maybe psychopathic/sadistic, and sometimes anger at the financial cost of feederism. In the UK, this is expressed through rage at the National Health Service (NHS) treating obese individuals, whilst in the U.S. it causes speculation that such individuals raise the cost of health insurance.

These factual depictions of feederism have inevitably been used and exaggerated to inform fiction. The Australian film "Feed" (2005) is an example of this. The film's plot focuses on two police officers who decide to investigate a heavily protected and secret feeding-fetish website featuring obese women. The site is shown having the kind of encryption normally associated with child pornography. When the owner of the website is tracked down, it transpires that the women on his site have been abducted and are deliberately being fed to death for the benefit of the website's owner and users. By the end of the film it is apparent that the owner of the website had a disturbed childhood and murdered his own obese mother.

DOI: 10.1057/9781137470461.0005

The portrayal of feederism in this film is an exaggeration of the already extreme mainstream depictions. "Feed" represents feederism as a fetish in which coercion takes place that is synonymous with domestic violence and suggests that it has developed from an unhealthy family situation. It is presumed that the fetish developed from an earlier pathology. Michael (the feeder), who is holding women captive in his cabin, is the prototypical feeder in the mainstream. He is someone who has nefarious intentions and someone who is ultimately in need of psychological treatment. A closer scrutiny of the feederism community paints a different story.

The ways in which the media has chosen to explore feederism has been to focus on the most extreme end of the subculture. In doing so it has enabled and legitimized a kind of voyeurism and criticism which otherwise appears unseemly or cruel. Being confronted with a sexualized fat woman such as Gina or Simpson (or fictional characters) allows the viewer to look at, and voice their disgust of, the fat female body in a way which may normally seem unacceptable. Fat women are invisible in Western society (Murray, 2004, 2008). They are not seen as sexual beings, and they are viewed as failures and morally weak. Fat women are seldom seen on television or in films except as devices for humour or to be pitied (the excruciating film "Shallow Hal" is the epitome of this (Burstein, 2001)). They are rarely seen in conventional women's magazines unless their image accompanies a success story of becoming thin. To desire a fat woman is deviant because to be desirable is to be thin. To be fat is to adopt a stigmatizing role.

Psychological research

Given the response of the general public and the media to feederism, it is surprising that there has not been more psychological research on this subculture. Lesley Terry is one of the few psychologists who has published specifically in the area of feederism rather than fat fetishism. Analysing Terry's (2007) thesis on "Food, Feeding, and Female Sexual Arousal," along with the articles (Terry & Vasey, 2011; Terry, Suschinsky, Lalumiere, & Vasey, 2012) that developed from it, provides a detailed picture of the limited published psychological perspective on this topic. Terry provides a brief cross-cultural context for the status of fat women in Western society by highlighting that the modern Western beauty ideal of a svelte woman is atypical if a global perspective on beauty is taken.

DOI: 10.1057/9781137470461.0005

Larger women are seen as preferable to slim women, particularly in African countries such as Mauritania and Nigeria. LaFraniere (2007) describes Mauritanian fattening huts where women are sent before marriage to be fattened. Women almost immobilized by fat are seen as an ideal in Mauritania, and LaFraniere outlines the over-feeding process: "Girls as young as five and as old as 19 had to drink up to five gallons of fat-rich camel's or cow's milk daily" (p.1). If girls resisted this practice or vomited they were tortured by the village "weigh gain specialist." Although the practice of torture is in decline, deliberate over-feeding of young girls and women is still common. Appearing slim can lead to being regarded as poor and therefore undesirable. As the human *gavage* aspect of this ideal recedes, LaFraniere reports an increase in the sale of pharmaceuticals designed to encourage weight gain (e.g. steroids and antihistamines). Thompson (2014) highlights how the disabling levels of obesity admired in Mauritania effectively exclude women from taking part in their communities or being involved in politics. She also adds that overweight girls will have early onset puberty and therefore appear more mature and with longer reproductive potential than their thinner counterparts, thus allowing earlier marriage (Kaplowitz (2008) reviews a number of articles linking body fat in girls with pubertal onset and suggests that weight gain may explain the falling age of menarche seen over the last 150 years across the U.S. and Europe). Thompson suggests that the fatness of young women serves to meet the needs of their husbands by making them look wealthy and allowing greater reproduction. This fattening tradition of *leblouh* has been covered in numerous women's magazines and often in great detail (e.g. Haworth, 2011), as it presents such sharp contrast to what is typically considered desirable in Western culture.

Larger women are also preferred within the fat-admiration communities of Western cultures. Fat admiration has been fully accepted by the National Association to Advance Fat Acceptance (NAAFA) as normal and to be encouraged. Essentially the position of NAAFA is that men and women of size who find each other attractive and want to form relationships should not be stigmatized, but the NAAFA has refused to support a subculture which finds weight *gain* erotic.

In many ways psychology has also sought to pathologize feederism. Terry (2007) suggests that feederism is a paraphilia by demonstrating how it meets the DSM-IV-TR (APA, 2000) criteria of unusual activities of attraction and unusual objects of attraction. Consulting the more

DOI: 10.1057/9781137470461.0005

recent DSM-5 (APA, 2013), it is certainly clear that feederism fits with the description of a paraphilia: "The term *paraphilia* denotes any intense and persistent sexual interest other than sexual interest in genital stimulation or preparatory fondling with phenotypically normal, physically mature, consenting human partners" (DSM-5, p.685). The sexual arousal experienced by feeders and feedees relates to the act of feeding and to weight gain. The sexual focus appears to be clearly on the food and its potential effects even though conventional sex may follow the feeding and eating. Many pieces of feederism fiction culminate with conventional sexual relations even though much of the story has focused on the food and the sensations of fullness experienced by the feedee or the effects of their size (e.g. bursting clothes, trouble exercising). Personal ads for feeders and feedees also focus very much on the potential for growth rather than sex.

The DSM-5's keenness to distinguish paraphilia from paraphilic disorders is important here. A paraphilic *disorder* is "a paraphilia that is currently causing distress or impairment to the individual or a paraphilia whose satisfaction has entailed personal harm, or risk of harm, to others" (DSM-5, pp.685–686). To label feederism as a paraphilic disorder seems excessive when one considers the willingness and apparent enjoyment of participants, and the fact that many engage in feederism far below the level of feeding to immobility or force-feeding. However, an argument could be made that extreme feederism meets the criteria for paraphilic disorder based on the harm to the feedee (despite his/her consent to be fed). Terry suggests that feederism may be most appropriately placed in the category of sadomasochism when trying to classify it as a paraphilia. In addition to the master-slave dynamic of the feeder-feedee, Terry (2007) also points to the preponderance of females in the feedee role, which parallels the high numbers of women involved in masochism compared to any other type of paraphilia.

Whilst it is interesting and potentially useful to consider feederism as a paraphilia or paraphilic disorder, it offers little insight into the deeper psychology behind the behaviour. Journalists and members of the public have been eager to speculate on the psychological dynamics of feederism relationships, whilst psychologists themselves have rarely contributed to the discussion. Terry (2007, 2011) explores the case of a self-identified feedee named Lisa and provides a rare exploration of the life history of someone sexually aroused by feederism. In her teens, Lisa was underweight, with a BMI of 16–18 and followed a strict diet of restricting her

DOI: 10.1057/9781137470461.0005

food to keep thin. She reports enjoying the sense of control that this gave her. Once her family became concerned, her overweight mother took control of her eating to ensure that she ate larger amounts. Despite being thin in her early teenage years, Lisa reports a fascination with fat from the age of seven or eight and sexual arousal to images of fat women from the age of 13. At the time of being interviewed, Lisa indicated that her arousal to images of fat women had become more specific, and she now became "aroused by seeing changes in a woman's body as she gained weight" (Terry, 2007, p.24).

As the case study of Lisa unfolds, it becomes clear why Terry feels that feederism may be appropriately placed into the category of sado-masochism. Lisa describes how she fantasizes about being ridiculed and humiliated for her weight gain (e.g. being called "fatty") and also how she would like to be fed by a dominant male who becomes aroused by her weight gain (Terry, 2007). She further indicates that she finds it difficult to have an orgasm unless she is fantasizing about feederism activity. Over a four month period Lisa claims to have engaged in a kind of autoerotic feederism where she purposefully increased her weight by 35 lbs for sexual pleasure. She documented this process with photographs and measurements. Lisa's weight gain has limits because she is concerned about the health consequences of becoming obese. If there were no health risks, she would like to be in the obese class II range (a BMI of 35 or more) but not to be immobile.

Lisa describes herself as having a real self and a feedee self (Terry, 2007). Her real self is fairly critical and unsympathetic towards overweight people and displays anti-fat attitudes. Her feedee self is the version of her which is happy to gain weight and become aroused by it. Terry (2007) explores a psychoanalytic perspective on Lisa and concludes that she does not really fit with the Freudian idea of oral fixation. Lisa has not experienced obvious trauma which could have triggered her feederism, nor does she enjoy the process of eating for itself. Lisa does not report finding tastes, textures, and aromas of food arousing, but simply the idea of weight gain. Terry theorizes that Lisa's behaviours and desires are a thematic variation on masochism and represent a form of Escape From Self based on Baumesiter's theory of masochism (Baumeister, 1988).

Baumeister does not pathologize masochism in the way that the DSM does, but instead regards it as a method to escape from higher-level thinking and awareness. He links this with the notion of the "burden

DOI: 10.1057/9781137470461.0005

of selfhood." Baumeister documents several studies and examples showing how common masochism is and how those who engage in it can be "normal" successful people (e.g. "among prostitutes catering to rich and powerful clients in Washington D.C., requests to be beaten outnumber requests to inflict beatings about eight to one" (Baumeister, 1988, p.32)). Incidences of masochism are hard to find until the 18th century, which coincides with a cultural change in Western societies that began to favour individualism. Earlier descriptions of apparently masochistic behaviour are limited to religious contexts rather than sexual ones. Baumeister advances these observations to support his theory that modern pressures of individualism and autonomy lead to masochism as a way to escape. Crushing self-awareness either through physical or emotional pain forces an individual to focus on the here and now and liberates them from thinking about consequences. It is conceivable that some aspects of feederism remove the burden of selfhood by giving control to the feeder and also by allowing the feedee to disavow mainstream cultural messages about being thin and in control.

This can be seen by the popularity in the feederism community of the 1937 *Merrie Melodies* cartoon called "Pigs is Pigs." A number of the interviewees for the present research spontaneously mentioned this cartoon, and others were aware of it when prompted. Those who mentioned it spontaneously described enjoying the cartoon and having a sort of fascination with it. One interviewee reported that the cartoon served as an inspiration for other artwork, fantasies, and other types of fiction. The cartoon lasts for seven minutes and 25 seconds, and the central character is Piggy Hamhock. Piggy is imprisoned by a slim, "evil scientist" who has constructed a large array of mechanisms designed to force-feed him. Piggy is restrained in a chair and rendered immobile with a device that opens and closes his mouth (while holding his nose) to allow food in and to force him to swallow. Piggy is propelled by the scientist's equipment through a basement factory where he is confronted with countless devices that force food into his mouth. There is a machine which mixes several varieties of soup before a rotating spoon shovels them into Piggy's mouth, a mechanized hand pushes bananas into his mouth and the same hand works a coin-operated olive feeder, bellows blow balls of ice cream at him, and Piggy is then launched towards a huge sausage and mustard sandwich while his mouth is moved up and down as though he were a machine. Many other examples follow, all showing Piggy looking frightened and totally at the mercy of the scientist as food is forced into

DOI: 10.1057/9781137470461.0005

him. As the cartoon closes Piggy is seen to have grown dramatically and his restraints can barely hold him. The scientist prods his spherical body and asks, "Had enough, my boy?" Piggy answers "Yes, sir," and as he's released, the scientist comments "Why, you're not even half full" as Piggy waddles past him towards the door. As Piggy is leaving, he walks past a large table of food. He looks longingly at it, and then eagerly picks up and eats a chicken leg shortly before exploding. Piggy wakes up screaming in his bed showing that the whole thing has been a dream. His mother calls him for breakfast and he rushes downstairs only to resume eating as fast as possible.

The cartoon clearly shows some elements of the extremes of feederism. The scientist as feeder has recognized Piggy's desire to eat and exploits that by stuffing him to the point of explosion. He has designed specialized equipment both to feed and restrain. Piggy, though restrained, is a willing participant as evidenced by his decision to keep eating after getting his freedom even though he is greatly swollen and barley able to walk. What is interesting is that this cartoon held a fascination for some interviewees before puberty and before any sexualization of weight gain had occurred. Pigs is Pigs also inspired an artist called Willix. Willix posts his work on Deviant Art and calls it Pigs *Be* Pigs [emphasis added]. He is open about basing his drawings on the 1937 cartoon and the cover of his comic states "a fantastic tale of force feeding and massive weight gain. Adapted from the 1937 Merrie Melodies short 'Pigs is Pigs'" (Pigs Be Pigs, 2008). Willix depicts a similar storyline to the original cartoon but with a woman in place of Piggy. There is also more obvious sexuality in the Willix cartoon, with the scientist showing great appreciation for the fattening body he is creating. Willix also develops the story to include a second woman and the main character becoming a superhero. His other art is all centred on obese women of different races standing or sitting in different outfits. Mostly they are wearing t-shirts and trousers, but he sometimes depicts the women in bikinis or pyjamas. If males feature in his work, they are typically drawn as slim yet appreciative of the large woman. This connects to another reference made by one participant to the English nursery rhyme "Jack Sprat." First published in 1639, the brief rhyme is simply:

> Jack Sprat could eat no fat.
> His wife could eat no lean.
> And so between them both, you see,
> They licked the platter clean (Jack Sprat, 1639/2015).

DOI: 10.1057/9781137470461.0005

The participant felt this was an influence in very early childhood[1] and placed the idea of fat women in his mind. It is certainly common in some kinds of feederism fiction to find a slim (and therefore controlled) man doing the feeding.

Of interest in both the original cartoon and the later comic book version is the idea of forcing and what it really represents. The original cartoon makes it quite clear at the end that Piggy will keep stuffing himself even when he's freed, and he doesn't learn anything from his restraints and loss of power. In the comic book, the female character reveals very early on that she used to be 327 lbs., suggesting that at some point she has engaged in prolonged and significant overeating, so therefore, she may still have a propensity towards it. Eventually the female character announces that the scientist should "call the gym" because she's "quit," and she embraces overeating again. The message from the cartoons is that the scientist is simply mechanizing and fulfilling an existing desire in the recipient even though they resist at first.

In another psychological analysis, Terry et al. (2012) sampled members of the public who do not belong to any feederism-related community. Their sample comprised 15 men and 15 women with the purpose of testing the hypothesis that feederism is an exaggerated response to normal sexual arousal to food and feeding. Participants were shown sexual, neutral, and feeding still images while listening to audio recordings of sexual, neutral, and feeding stories. Terry et al. (2012) measured genital responses to each image and the narratives, and they found that participants did not respond genitally to feeding stimuli, but both men and women rated feeding stimuli as more sexually arousing than the neutral stimuli. Terry et al. state that food and sex have been inextricably linked for centuries and food has aphrodisiac qualities that have been culturally disseminated and discussed. Although there was no physiological response, food is seen as a precursor to sex, indicating that sexual arousal is imminent. Terry et al. therefore contextualize feeding as indicative of male provisioning, as those who could successfully provide food achieved greater reproductive success, which is an evolutionary perspective on the fattening involved in feederism.

In an article for *The Daily Telegraph*, Moore (2010) analysed two British women dabbling in feederism. The first woman, Lucy, engages in online feeding sessions through Fantasy Feeder. Lucy's feeder watches her through a webcam whilst she eats doughnuts, cake, and ice cream. The second, Jess, describes herself as an active gainer and either eats alone

DOI: 10.1057/9781137470461.0005

or is aided by members of Fantasy Feeder (Moore, 2010). Like Lisa in Terry's (2007) case study, Jess had long-standing fantasies about expanding and would imagine growing larger and larger as a child. Unlike Lisa, she doesn't see gaining as an act of submission but rather an act of rebellion. She regards it as challenging female beauty norms in the same way that not wearing makeup or not removing body hair does.

An anonymous article for the website xoJane (Anonymous, 2013) described the counterintuitive ways in which s/he embraced being fat and desiring to grow larger. It is seen as counterintuitive to other people because, according to the author, fat is feared or simply accepted rather than sought after. The author describes finding online forums which dispelled the idea that feederism is purely coercive and based on a gendered dynamic of the feedee being a passive victim fed by a dominant powerful man. S/he states, for example, "It rings pretty misogynistic to me to assume that a woman (feedees are typically, though not always, women) who might be into eating a lot of food and getting fat must be being 'tricked' into it" (Anonymous, 2013).

In finding this online community, the author describes how he/she had intellectual discussions alongside erotic conversations about the nature of fat, but this led to a dual life where secrecy played a significant role. There is a literal self and a fantasy self, whereby limitations are recognized in normal everyday living but are breached and sabotaged in the fantasy world.

Another way in which feederism can potentially be pathologized is through the idea of addiction. During two interviews a participant expressed a desire to stop engaging in feederism because he felt it was putting him at risk. A second interviewee also spoke about planning to stop overeating whilst engaging in binge eating, the idea being each time that the current binge would be the last. These experiences raise the question of whether feederism shares any of the characteristics of a conventional addiction, and if it does, whether that would allow some form of therapy or intervention to be developed for those wanting to stop. In recent years there has been a growing tendency to accept certain behaviours as addictions rather than restricting the term to alcohol and drugs (Thege et al., 2015). Whilst feederism has not been specifically considered before, related activities such as food addiction and sex addiction have.

There is no consensus on what causes and maintains addiction. The brain disease model of addiction (BDMA) is favoured by many medical

DOI: 10.1057/9781137470461.0005

professionals, psychologists, and governments, but it has recently come under some criticism (Hall, Carter, & Forlini, 2015). The BDMA posits that addiction is a physiological brain disease which causes neurochemical changes that are incredibly difficult to reverse. Brain circuitry involved in reward is "hijacked," and the addicted person is no longer able to make choices or refrain from addiction-related behaviours. This model has suited policy makers as it reduces the stigma associated with the idea that addicts are weak-willed individuals who *choose* to keep taking drugs. It also allows medical interventions to be used alongside legal sanctions. Evidence for the model comes from both animal studies and human neuroimaging research that shows "dopamine mediated changes in cortical areas" related to impulse control (ibid., p.106). The BDMA also incorporates genetic factors, which are thought to explain between 40% and 70% of the variance in addictive behaviours relating to substance use (Kendler et al., 2012). Kendler et al. (2012) comment that environmental factors are most important in the initiation of drug use, whereas genetic factors play a more significant role in the continuation of drug taking. Criticisms of the BDMA suggest that addicts have far greater control over their behaviour. This is evidenced by research showing that addicts will abstain from drug use for 24 hours for financial reward, that many addicts experience spontaneous recovery, and that animal models of addiction begin to break down when the animals are housed in enriched and social environments rather than being alone in a bare cage (Hall et al., 2015).

The BDMA has mostly been used to explain addictions that have a chemical component to them (e.g. nicotine, opiates) but medical models are also applied to behavioural addictions (e.g. gambling). The DSM 5 was the first DSM to specifically categorize behavioural addictions. The working group involved in this decision "supported a unified neurobiological theory of addictions, regardless of the specific addictive substances, substrates, or activities" (Rosenberg & Feder, 2014, p.1). If feederism is an addiction, it would probably be classified as a behavioural one, as this is how both sex and (controversially) food addiction are currently understood. Yau et al. (2014) question whether food should be seen more like a chemical addiction, particularly in those who binge eat, but this is currently resisted due to the potential implications of labelling some foods as "addictive." Food also poses difficulties in the addiction arena because eating (unlike drug or alcohol use) is essential. This makes the abstinence message that is common to many addiction

DOI: 10.1057/9781137470461.0005

treatments unworkable. Nevertheless, Yau et al. report analyses showing that energy-dense foods activate the same dopaminergic pathways as those seen in drug addicts.

The evidence for sex addiction is less clear than for other behavioural addictions. Rosenberg, O'Connor, and Carnes (2014) report that "there is little convincing data that currently demonstrates a neurobiological pathway for sex addiction" (p.225). Some evidence points towards a genetic component in dysfunctional sexual behaviour, but it is by no means as clear as the findings relating to other addictions. Given that feederism is a sexual activity and is not simply about uncontrollable eating, it is currently difficult to see how it could be reliably classified as addiction either chemically or behaviourally. In some ways, this may add to the stigma some people involved in feederism feel. Thege et al. (2015) investigated public attitudes towards different addictions and found that individuals with behavioural addictions (e.g. shopping and eating) were judged to be more morally weak and blameworthy than those who had chemical addictions (e.g. heroin) even though evidence from neuroscience now suggests that many addictions have the same underlying neurological mechanisms. These findings suggest that an individual with feederism is unlikely to receive sympathy and support even if it were possible to label them as an addict. It is also important to acknowledge that despite finding feederism uncontrollable at times, it may not be appropriate to consider it an addiction. Most people involved in feederism do not feel out of control. They also fail to report forms of emotional dysfunction and harm commonly associated with addiction. Just because behaviours and thoughts are sometimes ego-dystonic, it should not automatically render them potential addictions. The "addict" label may be another way for individuals to disown their "deviant" or stigmatizing choices.

Sociological research

This section critically considers the sociological literature that has engaged with feederism, such as the notion that it represents an act of patriarchy. Research that has looked at fat more broadly, and issues relating to body types and the role fat plays in a society that privileges thin bodies, is also analysed. Issues of stigmatized identity are considered, and the historical context of sexuality is briefly considered to challenge

DOI: 10.1057/9781137470461.0005

assumptions that have developed in the sociological work engaging with feederism.

The mainstream depictions of feederism easily generate interest and commentary as previously outlined because they show a sexuality that is "deviant" (obese women as desired) yet one which also conforms to heteronormative expectations placing the man in control of the woman. Feederism in its most simplistic element is more complicated than it may initially seem.

Sociologists have begun to look at food and the rituals and symbols around it as a frame (Goffman, 1974) for understanding "[...]what and who we are, to ourselves and to others which can reveal new ways of thinking about those relations" (Probyn, 2000, p.14). Rettie (2009) notes, "For Goffman, a frame is not merely an informational context, but an integral part of the shared experience of interaction, and consequently an essential analytical tool if we want to understand the interaction" (p.425). A frame is therefore a way of viewing the world and a way of conveying information. To understand the context of meanings, it is important to look at how the issue is being framed. As a concept, this will be explored further in this section as a way of examining how 1) the previous academic literature has viewed feederism sociologically and 2) how other analysis might fit into the discussion by expanding the focus. Other studies have used framing as a way to look explicitly at the idea of how fat is presented as a general concept (Saugy, 2013), and this will be looked at in detail to see if feederism can fit into the prescribed frames that already exist.

The most cited sociological piece of work looking at feederism is a master's thesis by Bestard (2008). The study was exploratory and looked at analysing the experiences of 30 heterosexual respondents with a particular interest in how stigmatization factored into feederism as a lifestyle choice and how stigma was coped with. The research was the first attempt at conducting an empirical investigation and focused on the following research questions: "What is feederism? How is it defined and practiced by those who are interested in it?" (ibid., p.2). Bestard applied symbolic interactionism as a theoretical framework to understand the socially constructed meanings that feederism has for individuals. Symbolic interactionism is a theory that builds on three central assumptions: "(a) people strive and act toward what represents meaning for them, (b) meaning arises out of social interaction, and (c) meaning is being dealt with and modified through interpretive processes" (Handberg

DOI: 10.1057/9781137470461.0005

et al., 2014, p.1). It is therefore a good theoretical tool for looking at different types of meaning and significance that each participant felt for their sexual preferences for erotic weight gain. Another frame used by Bestard (2008), which was a successful way of incorporating cultural elements into the analysis, was applying insights from Goffman's (1963) understanding of stigma.

Goffman (1963, p.3) describes a stigma as an attribute such as a perceived character flaw that is regarded as "deeply discrediting" by other people in society. Having these attributes means potentially having a "spoiled identity." A person with a spoiled identity is often isolated from society, and in our new digitalized world, this means that they often find themselves feeling more comfortable expressing themselves online (Castells, 1996). The significance of the online space for dealing with stigma will be discussed later in this chapter. Bestard (2008) notes rightly that Goffman's work has been applied to a huge variety of different social issues, communities and individuals but that the explicit focus of combining stigma and feederism was a novel contribution. The most pertinent application of stigma has been to recognize that stigma permeates every facet of social life and as such affects issues such as family and interpersonal relations, employment opportunities, general wellbeing and everyday life itself. Feederism could be viewed as a type of stigma because having a sexual desire which sexualizes the deliberate gaining of weight for pleasure, is discrediting due to commonly accepted norms and values about beauty and health that permeate our culture (Walter, 2010). These stigmas are socially constructed in that they have a specific social base and context to them. Stigma operates at both the micro and macro level. O'Brien (2011, p.2) notes that cultural and political processes come together to create a link between "certain identifications and stigmatizing stereotypes," which is situated in a historical period and location.

The link between stigmatization and fat has been established for a long time and was evident only a few years after Goffman first published his text on stigma. An early example is Cahnman (1968) who looked at the implicit knowledge structures held in terms such as "obesity," "fat" and "overweight." The terms are what Bestard (2008, p.10) refers to as value-laden. The terms we use to describe overweight people are already tainted by various connotations which are conditioned by the type of society we have. There have been calls to reclaim these forms of terminology and so terms like fat have been placed in a similar context

DOI: 10.1057/9781137470461.0005

as the word queer has in forms of queer theory. The power of framing and discourse therefore is significant sociologically to how people who self-identity as a member of the feederism community feel about and choose to express themselves.

Bestard (2008, p.6) notes that her respondents felt feederism was "a sexual practice, a fetish, a sexual identity, a lifestyle, a fantasy, a subculture, and it has an online community." The community is linked to the idea of being part of what Goffman (1963) refers to as the own, which refers to a group of stigmatized individuals who are able to come together to reflect on their own stigmatization. The theoretical point made by Goffman was obviously more pertinent during the time he wrote stigma as online deviancy is more common-place and widely acknowledged now.

A pertinent issue is how we are expected to be good citizens in a neoliberal society (Tischner, 2013). This narrative frames the general discussion on feederism both explicitly or implicitly because it is an unchallenged assertion. We are encouraged to conform to healthy diets and regularly exercise as a way to maintain a socially sanctioned body type. To have a certain body type presupposes success, and to deviate from it means morally failing. Encouragement to conform to a specific body shape comes from various different interconnecting facets of the media. Different types of lifestyle almost seem inconsistent with the value-laden mantras associated with neoliberalism, which encourages a specific type of lifestyle where exercise and a healthy diet are prerequisites to a good life. The doctrine of free choice and agency is highly policed by acceptable ways of presenting your body (ibid.). A useful metaphor used by a number of different authors to discuss fat bodies is applying the concept of the panopticon building on the work of Foucault (1977). The panopticon was a hypothetical prison which allowed a single watchman to observe all the prisoners in an institution without them being aware that they were being watched. The implicit narratives that surround healthy bodies and individual choice acts as a type of social panopticon and means that different types of sexual identity such as feederism are hidden due to social pressures; being fat is associated with death and as a result fatness is framed as an omen for future disease and suffering (Tischner, 2013).

Body size and weight can be highly gendered issues because looking is not simply a passive act, there is a "discursive nature of in/visibility" (ibid., p.44). What is visible is a type of social process that is socially

DOI: 10.1057/9781137470461.0005

and internationally constructed; sexuality with regards to feederism has clear visual elements. The fat body has two distinct forms of surveillance surrounding it and as such another application of the panopticon metaphor is the idea of the body as being the site for the panopticon more generally. The body is under constant watch and so Germov and Williams (1999) discuss the notion of a body panopticon. It is a useful metaphor in discussing the ways in which the body is policed from multiple different frames. Tischner (2013, p.53) notes that "being slim is a socially constructed signifier of feminine beauty and of being heterosexually attractive as a woman in contemporary society."

Given all these forms of surveillance, it is interesting the extent to which feederism can be considered a deliberate breach of socially sanctioned body types. Diane, a participant in our research, described feederism as an act of rebellion, as a way of thwarting what she saw as deliberate sanctions on her expression of her own body and her own sexuality. Based on these observations, feederism may adequately fulfil the theoretical description of what constitutes a "body project" (Shilling, 2003). In feederism, the body is modified and perfected through eating excessive amounts of food, and it's a process that is never completed. It is a meticulous project, and weight gain is often monitored with the entire process almost being a parody of the contemporary diet, which focuses on calorie counting and weighing oneself on a daily basis. Foucault noted that there are certain "technologies of the self" available to people in expressing their identity and feederism is no different. It is a process that has fantasized elements as well as tangible expressions as noted previously when discussing Terry's (2007) case study of Lisa. A point of departure is that the body project is never entirely complete in the same way that tattoos, piercings or other body modification projects often are (Featherstone, 2000) and it is the process of feeding and getting larger which is the real erotic focus, the gradual expanding and stretching of the body. This deliberate and often meticulously calculated growth of the body is seen as atypical, harmful and thus a potentially deviant sexual behaviour (Bestard, 2008; Prohaska, 2013). The extent to which this is atypical, harmful and different is contested within our participants and within the academic literature. Featherstone (2000) notes that body projects are attempts at creating a concrete self-identity which is corporally focused. Modifying the body is an expression of the self, and in many ways, a chance to be different in a society that increasingly lives on change (Bauman, 1992). We have become a culture that is heavily

DOI: 10.1057/9781137470461.0005

focused on the thin body to such an extent that the photographs we see of celebrities and of people in the media in our magazines and newspapers are often modified to look a specific way, or to highlight a specific feature. These discourses are not the norm historically.

Historically there are conflicting accounts of how body image and sexuality coincided. Brumberg (2000) for example noted that in Victorian bourgeois society, eating was not indicative of individualized taste buds for young girls and women but rather a reflection of personality or individual character traits. With appetite becoming a social tool, frailty eventually became emphasized over indulgence, especially foods that have sensual properties like meat and candy. Certain foods were associated explicitly with sexuality and were therefore discouraged, especially for respectable women. This narrative of self-mastery is still a major discourse today with dieting regimes representing control and obesity with overabundance and fecklessness (Hester, 2009).

Other sources offer differing accounts of the larger body type. Jutel (2005) cites a source in the early 20th century (Wood & Rudduck, 1923) which identifies thin women as the type of woman that men should avoid when deciding on the qualities that their life partner should have. These attitudes were common in the media as well, which viewed the gaunt, svelte body as suspect. Jutel (2005) states that this is because these women were seen as man-haters with a lack of sexuality, which was apparently displayed by "flat chests, narrow hips, bloodless and thin or peaked features and a lack of warmth and softness that attracts and holds the affections of men" (Wood & Rudduck, 1923, p.861). The thin body was therefore implicated in a highly gendered discourse which viewed it within the social conditions at that time as being negative for femininity. Thin bodies were seen as being prone to disease, and young people were encouraged in particular to gain weight to avoid this. The narrative of health therefore switched from being focused on the failures of the thin body, to focusing on the fat body. Previously, being fat was lauded, particularly as a desirable feminine attribute in early holiday postcards that depicted women getting larger as a result of her holiday, or men encouraging women to gain weight. The men in the images are depicted as unrealistically skinny. Fat was therefore more likely to be seen as a feminine attribute, and so the very idea of what constitutes femininity has radically changed over time. Equally it could be noted that masculinity has also changed over time. The masculine body is nondescript and often minimized in order to accentuate the large female body in the

DOI: 10.1057/9781137470461.0005

holiday postcards mentioned. A repository of these images is available on the *Dimensions Magazine* website.

When looking at the issue of framing, Saugy (2013) culminated a decade long exploration of the question, "what's wrong with fat?" with a book outlining the various ways in which fat can be viewed or medicalized with terms such as "obesity." An area of interest is the outlining of "problem frames" (ibid., p.30) and how these existing structural frames might help to understand current trends within feederism. Viewing a discourse like this is powerful because it allows an examination of the commonly accepted socially constructed values (doxa) that underpin and uphold each theme. Analysing data like this can fill significant gaps in building the meanings behind the constructs, what Foucault referred to as a genealogical method.

Saugy (2013) outlined six typological categories which are: immorality, medical, public health crisis, Health at Every Size, beauty and fat rights. Feederism crosses all six of these. The problem frame depends entirely on who is being asked the questions. Saugy (2013) is aware that power is a significant factor here with different forms of capital at work across each and conceptualizes the notion of a "fat field" to recognize different symbolic or economic forms of capital across the main players in each field. Saugy (2013) has also noted that the bodily capital of the researchers involved in fat studies is significant, whereby thin researchers are taken more seriously as thin is an "unmarked category" (p.36), thin is not seen as having a body size or shape, it just is. This ultimately shows that fat is regarded generally as a pathogen, a "moral failing." This deconstructed complexity shows how vital the concept of a fat field is in recognizing these points. Feederism has a marginalized role within this field and is controversial due to its deviant status. The mainstream media has focused on immobility, a subset of feeding identification often associated with fantasies that quite clearly falls within an immoral framework. The behaviour is there for consumers to reject and label as inappropriate or scandalous, so reactions will be focused within this singular frame, which is then generalized across the entire subculture. Those who classify as active participants within feederism will evoke the "beauty" frame instead, which asserts that fat is beautiful and the problem is that mainstream society has conflated beauty with thin, slender bodies.

Another point to complicate this discussion is sexuality more generally. As feederism is commonly seen as a deviant sexual interest or aberration, it is useful to trace the contradictions and establishment of the notion of

DOI: 10.1057/9781137470461.0005

sexuality as a concept. What does it mean for us to state that something is a normal sexuality? The way in which sexuality is understood has made it easy to be disgusted, or troubled by atypical sexual behaviours because we have established a manual that is reflected in what Bourdieu (1984) calls the "habitus." The habitus includes the values, mores and lifestyle choices that are unconsciously appropriated and taken for granted by an individual in society. Crossley (2013) has since developed this notion to consider the ways in which body size, shape and image can create values and understandings that are unconsciously accepted, by coining the term "body habitus." Pyle and Lowey (2009) state that we live in a culture that is disdainful of fat bodies due to the assumption that they "[...] A) *choose* to be different and socially unacceptable, (B) could change if they really wanted to or tried harder, and, therefore, (C) deserve the discrimination that they experience (Pyle and Lowey 2009:144). This is reminiscent of Foucault's notion of 'disciplining bodies.'" How have the roots of sexual nomenclature structured thinking about what sexuality is, and how has this affected deviancy is viewed?

Foucault (1985) notes that the term "sexuality" did not emerge until the 19th century, and its emergence within common parlance happened as part of a larger set of phenomena (e.g. the development of different strands of knowledge that provided a greater understanding of the body such as the biological mechanisms of reproduction). Sexuality as it is understood now coincided with the development and reincorporation of new and traditional norms and mores. It was the beginning of a more reflexive society where individuals were expected to express their experiences with reference to specific labels and "[...] assign meaning and value to their conduct, their duties, their pleasures, their feelings and sensations [;] their dreams" (Foucault, 1985, p.4). Individuals came to recognize themselves as an individual taking part in sexuality to which others could ascribe meaning and understanding to. Moralistic standards were adopted which regulated the ways in which individuals experienced their sexuality. Narratives were established that changed the ways in which sexuality was understood and created a taxonomy of not only acceptable behaviours, but identities too. Sexuality wasn't outlawed or prevented, but rather reconceptualized.

Sedgwick (1990) notes the framing of sexuality and the notion of what is heterosexual or homosexual, traces back to this time frame. Cantarella (1992) noted the ancient Greeks were mostly a bisexual civilization but they didn't use dualistic language to differentiate classes of sexuality

DOI: 10.1057/9781137470461.0005

as sex was about power. Power is how feederism is often understood particularly as an unequal patriarchal relationship founded on masochism. Power was very clear historically when it came to sex, as the roman poet Catullus (Catullus & Lee, 1991) points out explicitly in the 16th poem in the only surviving manuscript of his writing. He berates and diminishes the status of a social foe by labelling him as a "catamite," stating that he will sodomize him. Catamite meant an anal receiver and was associated with notions of submissiveness and weakness and was typically associated with younger boys. The association of power with sex has been a symbiosis that has taken place from time immemorial, but the dynamics of it have changed somewhat. Historically, power within a sexual relationship was predicated on social standing rather than predetermined social characteristics such as gender. Thus, the understanding of "patriarchal power" dynamics within sexual relationships is relatively recent, historically speaking. Various authors have attempted to use this understanding with specific reference to feederism, but power is difficult to discern in the feederism dynamic, for reasons we will establish.

Another issue is how the fat body is displayed and a way in which this has been looked at is through analysing pornography. Kipnis (1996) notes that pornography is often a repository for deviant acts that are disavowed in society as a whole, and so feeding as a transgressive sexualized behaviour emerges as a result of this cultural narrative. The pornography in feederism is often singular; it does not feature other people with autoerotic acts being recorded for mass consumption (e.g. overindulgent eating or menial everyday tasks (Kulick & Meneley (2005)). Bestard (2008) reminds us that these types of pornography are specific subgenres within a larger more expansive area of fat pornography that is more conventional, but nonetheless the erotic display of the body in feederism is through food entering the mouth.

Sociological studies of feederism

Academic research in the field of feederism has been affected by the patriarchal representation, which has consistently failed to look deeper into the feederism subculture. This narrow portrayal of feederism has suited researchers with a feminist agenda who wish to highlight the practice as misogynistic and harmful to women. It is true that there are cases of feederism that fit this notion and fiction writing on feederism

DOI: 10.1057/9781137470461.0005

websites that also support it. However, there are also many examples of women who advertise for feeders and express a wish to be fed to immobility; mutual gaining in which both partners agree consensually to erotic weight gain; female feeders who look for men to fatten up; autoerotic feeding and fantasy elements that cross into other sexual fetishes.

Prohaska (2013) notes in a content analysis the ways in which feederism can be considered a transgressive sexual behaviour. She concludes through her analysis that despite occasionally displaying these elements, it typically mimics "patriarchal sex" in the process. The beginning of the article describes communities online that are predicated on stigmatized behaviour and examples are provided such as "bug chasers" or "bestiality." Feederism is placed within a pigeon hole before the analysis can begin. The association with the pathological is implicit from its textual association. The article describes the ways in which the fat community and feminists have disagreed with feederism's transgressive potential and outlines the position taken by NAAFA. The position is as follows: "people of all sizes become empowered to demand respect for their bodies in the content of sexual relationships, without attempting to lose or gain weight in order to win a partner's approval or attract or retain that partner's desire" (cited in Prohaska, 2013, p.104). Interesting in this statement is the notion of respect for one's body. It seems apparent that "respect" for the body here has a moralizing discourse underlying it. The body can only be adequately respected if it maintains a particularized health narrative that is disavowed or outright rejected in the "feeding community." In discussing *docile bodies* Foucault (1973), noted how morality and medicine often overlap. Also implicit in this statement is that gaining or losing weight is done within a coercive power dynamic. The gaining body is only gaining in an effort to "win" the desire of a partner. The language used here is particularly striking; it is not a consensual dynamic where a partner is gaining in a consensual relationship where desire is shared. Desire is understood as a singular entity that is obtained or won like a prize by fulfilling a set of body obligations.

NAAFA dismisses the entire feederism community because of a belief that it is non-consensual and is predicated on unequal power relations. Being fat in general does have its share of social problems and pressures that might create stigmas that interrelate with other pre-existing inequalities (e.g. Pyle & Loewy (2009) note a "double stigma" in a social case study looking at a marginalized subculture of queer fat men and their male admirers. These men do not fit the standardized image of

DOI: 10.1057/9781137470461.0005

what constitutes a gay man firstly, and they also do not conform to the standardized body habitus, which is a thin and smart appearance). In feederism, stigma is universalized across sexual boundaries, there is no heterosexist discrimination because many of the acts being stigmatized are consensual "atypical" heterosexual sex. It is also a more blatant disregard for a health-obsessed culture. It is not merely a stigma of appearance (e.g. lacking a clear structure when it comes to eating); it is a deliberate breach and disregard for these notions.

Prohaska (2014) attempted to reframe feederism within a sexual deviance framework by doing a content analysis of web-based materials that discuss feederism. There were three sources to her data-collection methodology. The initial stage was exploratory and collected data from internet searches relating to feederism (her search terms were: feederism, feedee; feeder, feeding, force-feeding and erotic weight gain: Prohaska, 2014, p.266). This was a rhizomatic method in the sense that Prohaska (2014) also collected data from sources that were linked within other pages, eventually leading to data that did not appear in the original search. There is a problem here from the offset: that force-feeding is not entirely synonymous with feederism. This is an example of where narrow interpretations of the subculture have affected academic discourse. Force-feeding is certainly an aspect in extreme circumstances, but it is such a niche practice that to accumulate data from this search seems to assume certain power relationships from the offset, which are generalized to the entire sexual subculture. Indeed Prohaska (2014, p.268) herself notes that force-feeding was "[...] rarely discussed as a legitimate behaviour by community members" within her content analysis. Bestard's (2008) interview subjects also noted that this sort of extremism is a fringe element of an otherwise universally consensual sexual behaviour.

Prohaska's (2014) second data collection method applied Bestard's (2008) theoretical ideas interviewing members of the feederism community through email exchanges. Lastly, Prohaska analysed forum posts from Fantasy Feeder for three months. Fantasy Feeder featured forums offering support, advice and information on sexual practices, including photographs and entries describing "stuffing, belly inflation, and squashing" (Prohaska 2014, p.267). Advertising on the sites analysed directed users to visit dating and flirting sites designed exclusively for lovers of fat. What is notable is that Fantasy Feeder also features forums and pages for people interested in meeting up, and it covers all ages and sexes. Despite the brief mention of this data, the detail is lacking.

DOI: 10.1057/9781137470461.0005

A thorough content analysis is required, especially one that pertains to an understanding of the sexual behaviour as pathological or normative deviance. Despite this, numerous things can be derived from the content analysis offered. Feeders and encouragers tend to be male and gainers or feedees tend to be female. Prohaska (2014) noted that these relationships only rarely became abusive or coercive. The conclusion that is drawn from these insights is that feederism is a communal activity because members of the community benefit emotionally and practically from like-minded individuals (ibid.). Part of the problem with this assertion is that the sample presupposes such a conclusion. The content analysis was done using forums and sites that aim to provide advice and emotional support. As Prohaska (ibid.) notes herself, there are a number of behaviours that constitute feederism, and one of them is autoerotic feeding. The communal hypothesis suggests that the sexual acts that fall under the banner of feederism are only happening online or within groups, which could be mistaken. An important conclusion that Prohaska (ibid.) makes concerns the way in which mainstream society has rejected seemingly consensual sexual acts, due to preconceived notions of what constitutes a healthy body. A healthy body is not fat, and it is also one that is intensely reflexive about dieting and meticulous about eating "right." It is therefore important to look at how feederism can be understood in different ways using the theoretical literature available.

Unlike most literature on feederism, Murray (2004) looks at the intersections of sex and fat. She discusses the idea that fat women are culturally presented as being asexual and without desire and are not desired generally. She considers desire as a social construction as fat bodies are coded as representing or symbolizing a failed self. Murray (2004) discusses how being fat could act as a "defiant blockage" and therefore as a form of resistance. This links with Giddens' (1991) notion of a body project in that within postmodernity, we are increasingly using our bodies to express ideas, beliefs and identities that are malleable. It also links to Orbach's (1978) thesis in stating that sex is only occupied by "the normative thin female body" (Murray, 2004, p.240); many fat women desire to be thin in order to gain access to the sexual realm. Being fat avoids one's sexuality altogether. Mutual gaining feederism shows that fat can be sexualized, however, it could be stated that this realm of sexuality is a very specific thread and is carnivalesque rather than being universally regarded as sexual. Murray (2004, p.244) makes the point that many of the acts associated with fat acceptance are actually "reversing the dominant aesthetic

DOI: 10.1057/9781137470461.0005

ideal" instead of subverting or dismantling it. The presentation of the fat body is often done through the same objectifying lens that characterizes other body types. The problem Murray has outlined is that merely sexualizing fat women does not eradicate the underlying problems that are associated with the way we think of women's bodies in the first place. We therefore need a fat acceptance that does not reproduce the same underlying problems. Beautifying the fat body and sexualizing it for a male audience through empowerment therefore is not challenging the dominant knowledge structures that presuppose this as a normal way of presenting the body. An example of this can be seen in the weekly stripping event called "Thick Sundaes" in Las Vegas, Nevada, which aims to promote and celebrate fat bodies and showcase their sexuality through erotic dancing.

Murray (2004) presents a niche and somewhat sensationalized perspective of feederism that focuses on immobilization, which is a small and extreme part of the subculture. Feederism is not a distinctly asymmetrical, patriarchal dynamic, as men force-feeding women is only one dynamic out of other possible scenarios, such as homosexual feeding and male feedees. Murray's research is now a decade old, and much of the research conducted at the time only looked at and understood feederism from this very specific patriarchal dynamic.

Murray (2008) places the term fat within inverted commas because she challenges the notion that fat is "an empirical fact that in turn reveals a universalizing profile of the fat subject" (Murray, 2008, p.1). This is interesting because it challenges generalized cultural assumptions, such as the notion that the fat subject is lazy, not willing to change, is a compulsive eater or is hyper-emotional (ibid., p.4). Fat as a body type is a site for powerful discourses, what Bourdieu generally calls doxa (Bourdieu, 1984). Graham (2005) was aware of the ways in which our culture reads the fat body and coined the term "lipoliterates." The fat body is seen as a landscape onto an unhealthy lifestyle from which only death can result. Foucault (1973), in his notion of disciplinary medicine, noted that discourses are formed, which means that morality and medicine overlap. Probyn (2000 p.18) notes "[...]it is clear that food and eating is as much marked by pleasure as it is by power; in fact, it gestures to the pleasure of control, the desire revealed in constraint." Feederism is in a unique position here; the pleasure of control that Probyn notes is a pleasure of excess rather than constraint. The power at work here, then, is in disorienting standardized understandings of the body, health

DOI: 10.1057/9781137470461.0005

and what constitutes the sexy body in the mass media. Probyn also recognizes the intersection of eating and power. Feederism as a body project explicitly counters this line of thinking because it subverts and disorients the commonly accepted routes to fat. The moral distaste of fat is so ingrained that an alternative means to the established story becomes disorienting and difficult to comprehend. The sexualization of fat coinciding with the modification of the body or a partner's body to align with this eroticization disrupts the doxa.

In an earlier key text on the subject of feederism, Giovanelli and Peluso (2006) define feederism as the practice of "incorporating the eroticization of body fat and the act of feeding, along with discipline weight gain for participant's sexual gratification" (p.331). Engagement with feederism is done in a variety of different ways according to these authors, across the internet, fantasizing with partners. The definition used therefore is open-ended and allows for different types of experiences to be incorporated. The researchers set out to answer whether feederism was a fetish or a subculture where identities were re/formed as a result of sexual activity and behaviour. They were also interested in looking at what the practice of feederism means for dominant cultural norms and practices surrounding sexual behaviour and food more generally. They make theoretical distinctions between a fetish and subculture because how feederism is located in the academic literature affects the social, political and moral nuances of the individuals involved. "We acknowledge that feederism may encompass fetishistic behaviors, but we also believe that the individuals who participate in feederism may do so to challenge dominant norms surrounding sex and desirability – and members of subcultures are often afforded more political clout than are individuals invested in particular fetishes" Giovanelli and Peluso (2006, p.331).

The awareness in having more political poignancy when belonging to a subculture is seen as a pernicious underlying factor to the community, as if directly challenging dominant sexual norms was the primary objective of the subculture. As Bestard (2008) points out, Giovanelli and Peluso's (2006) work is purely theoretical and is not based on any empirical research data collection, and as they do not explain how they got their information on feederism, their insights here are purely speculative. With regards to being a fetish, the researchers refer to a theoretical analysis of female fetishism that is directly related to food, which recognizes the culturally constructed nature of the fetish (Gamman & Makinen, 1994). It is stated that due to the "culture of slenderness," fat bodies are seen as

DOI: 10.1057/9781137470461.0005

deviant, and so food has the same restrictions placed on it as sex does for many women. Both of these elements (food and sex) are "susceptible to dangerous and uncontrollable lusts" (Giovanelli & Peluso 2006, p.332). Eating is therefore an alternative way of achieving an orgasm for women. Particular foods are described as being more desirable, with healthier foods such as fruit and vegetables being ignored for foods which are more fattening. These types of food are more dangerous and more alluring and are seen as dangerous to a woman trying to maintain her femininity. The problem with the incorporation of this theoretical model of female fetishism and food is that it only looks at one particular gender within the Feederism community and thus assumes the standardized stereotypical image of gaining as being exclusively the domain of the woman. It also wrongly assumes that feederism eschews particular types of food in order to arrive at a larger body quicker as it ignores members of the community who eat a whole range of foods. Many members of the feederism community value the taste of the food they are consuming, and so whilst ultimately the food is a means to an end, the food taken is enjoyed and appreciated. Given all these points, it is not sufficient to link the culture of slenderness with a fetish for larger bodies, as a more intersectional approach is required which takes into consideration different types of masculinity and different types of sexualities such as gay mutual gaining versus straight heterosexual feedee/feeder relationships.

Giovanelli and Peluso (2006) describe different levels of commitment within the feederism community in what they term "lifestyle versus fantasising." Lifestyle feederism involves the incorporation of feederism into everyday relationships. The authors claim that there are many who simply fantasize and do not incorporate this, usually for practical reasons. This distinction is too simplistic, as often there is significant overlap with many who practice feederism in their everyday lives having fantasies that they recognize as not tenable due to other commitments. One of these fantasies is immobility, which is recognized as a fantasy construct. It also depends entirely on the sample and what the focus of the sample is, since there are a number of different roles that are common in the feederism community. Because no sample was taken by the authors in question, their conclusions are not grounded in data and therefore do not carry the same weight as other analyses.

There has been significant work in feminist studies on the issue of fat more broadly, and some of these key texts will be discussed briefly. In *Fat is a Feminist Issue*, Orbach (1978) radically conceptualized fat as not

DOI: 10.1057/9781137470461.0005

being the consequence of societal stereotypes such as laziness, but rather a challenge to gendered assumptions about femininity. Her work was regarded as an anti-dieting manifesto. Orbach's (1978) central point was that fat is a sometimes a deliberate (or unconscious) transgressive behaviour undertaken to avoid the commoditization of the body in an unequal patriarchal society. Women use "fat" as a way to protect themselves from sexuality (or "patriarchal sex" as Prohaska (2013) notes). Being fat offers a woman a buffer between corporeal commodification, such as unrealistic standards of beauty, and wider social inequalities, which Orbach (1978) argues is a systemic and historically persistent inequality; this is in line with standard theories of patriarchy (Walby, 1990). Part of the problem with this thesis is the way in which desire is conceptualized. Orbach's (1978) assertion is that women un/consciously become fat as a means to avoid desire altogether. One aspect that is particularly contentious for the purposes of this book is the notion that fat is synonymous with asexuality or an avoidance of desire. Feederism is a singular example which provides a real life subcultural case study to reject this. The *raison d'etre* for feeding is to provoke and stimulate desire. It is unique in the sense that the very process itself provokes erotic fixation, such as the swelling of the stomach. Fat is a feminist issue and can be an issue for provoking serious challenges to the standardized notions of beauty in society, but the reason that Orbach's (1978) thesis is inadequate is her operationalization of fat. Fat can be a way to actually engage with sexualization and a way to explore the body in new ways.

There has been concern that women enter relationships with men not knowing they are feeders and as such it can lead to a domestic-violence dynamic. This does not seem to be backed up through empirical data. The sentiments are generally quite misleading if they are generalized to the entire sexual fetish and might be a failed attempt at constituting a moral panic (Cohen, 1972). We can see this if we look at the forums and stories that are common within the feederism subculture, where forced elements are more niche, and consensual sexual dynamics are more common. A key problem in the literature thus far has been to ignore or to avoid covering the ways in which women can take an active role in a feederism sexual dynamic. An example is female feedees acting in a more dominant role, or a female feeder dominating a submissive male feedee.

Although previous research (Murray, 2004; Prohaska, 2013) has focused on the female feedee and the male feeder, the current research

DOI: 10.1057/9781137470461.0005

attempts to consider the myriad of possibilities available when these roles are challenged, and the diversity of sexuality is taken into account. We also seek to challenge another common misconception that has been assumed in the published academic literature which is that feederism relationships seek to produce immobility in one of the parties. This is a potential dramatic conclusion, but it is not the norm.

As implicitly asserted by many authors looking at feederism, it is a communal activity that is documented and digitalized. Much of the research so far looking at feederism has used the internet as a tool for recruitment and for ascertaining information generally about what constitutes feederism. As Hakim (2015, p.315) notes, the distinction between private/solo sexual activities and partnered social activities are eroding. These distinctions, which previously meant that more arcane and niche forms of sexuality were hidden from view, have changed due to the digitalized ways in which we interact now. Another important point that Hakim (ibid.) make is that sexuality straddles the fence between physiology, sociology and the public/private. Sexuality is also being framed by the prevailing digitalized culture we find ourselves in as Bauman (2003) has noted when discussing the idea of "liquid love."

The digitalized culture is not problematic for sampling purposes. As Gies (2008) notes in his discussion of *cyber-bodies*, the demarcated gap between the online and offline world is becoming increasingly tenuous. The definition of *offline* might need to change with an omnipresent fast speed internet connection being the norm. It does alter the assumptions that were traditionally held about sexual identities, though, because the digital world ontologically might have an impact on how these identities are expressed and shared, as hinted at by theorists who look critically at the changing nature of modernity like Bauman. Gies (2008, p.312) notes in direct opposition to notions held in postmodernism about the elusive and free-floating lack of stability when it comes to expressing or having an identity, that "[...] material bodies reinforce their presence on the internet." Mongahan (2005) comments that subcultural identities are incentivized to group together online as a way to share pleasures, discomforts and information relating to their everyday lives. O'Brien (2011) discusses the ways in which individuals who carry a common stigmatized identity can learn about and practice ways to manage their spoiled identity together in private, what Goffman (1959) refers to as the "back stage." This way of managing a

DOI: 10.1057/9781137470461.0005

spoiled identity is particularly prevalent with people involved in feederism, who often band together on forums, creating online communities offering encouragement, advice and a space to communicate about all aspects of feederism.

These arguments provide an interesting contrast to theoretical developments within feminist theory. Within cyber-feminist perspectives, there is a notion that woman's liberation can take place digitally due to users online not being limited to social constraints such as having the wrong gender or having the wrong race (Morohan-Martin, 2000). Two perspectives are called into question: First, the cyber-feminist position outlined is unrealistic and does not take into consideration how subcultures actually use the internet. Secondly, what Prohaska (2014, p.104) calls "dystopian cyber feminists" is also debatable. This theoretical school argues that users online will be constrained by their offline identities, stating that norms are fluid. As discussed, the dichotomous notion of offline/online needs to be challenged, and thus it is not useful to assume either position. In effect, both positions have a grain of truth to them, and this will become even more apparent when two things happen with the internet. The first is a drive to secrecy, security and anonymity in the face of excessive government surveillance, but secondly, the globalization of networks and the democratization of the internet across the world. Given this nuance, it is bizarre how many academics have viewed the interrelationship between feederism as a sexual identity/body project and the use of the internet (e.g. Prohaska (2013, p.104) "In turn, research has not concluded if the internet is liberating women of size, or if it is just another form of patriarchal sex"). Patriarchal sex is nebulous because it groups any form of heterosexual sex that is consensual (or non-consensual). It is sex with the ultimate goal of conquest, which for Prohaska covers all consensual heterosexual relationships. It is clear from the feederism community that different types of feeding identities and relationships exist, particularly transgressive groupings that include mutually gaining men. It also does not disqualify the sexual behaviour from being transgressive simply because it is heterosexual. Indeed, if the dynamics were reversed, and the feeding relationship was between a man who was being fed by his domineering female partner, it would still have the makings of patriarchal sex for Prohaska, since ultimately the man's desires are the desires being fulfilled first and foremost.

DOI: 10.1057/9781137470461.0005

Conclusions

The methodologies used within the literature explicitly examining feederism have focused on conducting small-scale content analyses of forums, stories and artwork posted online, and have used interviews that were conducted by email. Real-time interviews with members of the feederism community reflecting on their experiences have not been published before. The literature published so far has developed some very useful tools and theoretical ideas, which we have combined with other research areas for nuance. Work has also been done looking at the stigmatization involved in having a "feeding identity," which has usefully applied theories developed by Goffman and other key sociological theorists (Bestard, 2008).

There has been useful work looking at the feederism community itself (Giovanelli & Peluso, 2006) and distinguishing between different levels of commitment in the community. These differences are something that has emerged in the current research with different levels of engagement with different types of sexual identity and varying levels of weight gain. These levels of commitment vary in fantasies as well, and so this work has been useful in providing a blueprint of diversity. Work looking at feederism through the lens of feminist theory has been useful in outlining power dynamics and the possibility of coercive relationship dynamics. The key problem with this work has been its limited focus, which presupposes specific gendered roles. The male is typically cast as the feeder and the female is cast as the feedee which ultimately frames power relations in a specific way. We think the feminist work that has been developed could be theoretically richer with a focus on different types of sexualized identity in feederism, particularly female feeders and male gainers.

The next chapter shows our research contribution to the field, addressing some of the gaps that have been outlined, particularly in exploring the diversity of the feederism community through a variety of different research methods. We have combined online analysis of stories with real-time voice interviews and written responses. The research that follows also offers a heuristic tool for future research and presents an extensive analysis of the experiences of people involved within this subculture.

Note

1 He also makes reference to the story of Hansel and Gretel where the children were encouraged to fatten up by eating a gingerbread house.

DOI: 10.1057/9781137470461.0005

References

American Psychiatric Association (2000). *Diagnostic and Statistical Manual of Mental Disorders* (4th ed., text revision). Washington, DC: APA.

American Psychiatric Association (2013). *Diagnostic and Statistical Manual of Mental Disorders* (5th ed.). Washington, DC: APA.

Anonymous (2013). *It Happened to Me: I Have a Sexual Fetish for Being Fed and Gaining Weight.* Retrieved February 5, 2015, from http://www.xojane.com/sex/weird-controversial-sexual-fetish-known-as-feedism.

Bauman, Z. (1992). *Intimations of Postmodernity* (1st ed.). London: Routledge.

Bauman, Z. (2003). *Liquid Love: On the Frailty of Human Bonds.* Polity Press: Cambridge.

Baumeister, R. F. (1988). Masochism as Escape from Self. *The Journal of Sex Research*, 25, 28–59.

Bestard, A. (2008). Feederism: An Exploratory Study into the Stigma of Erotic Weight Gain. Unpublished master's thesis, submitted for a master's degree, University of Waterloo, Waterloo, Ontario, Canada.

Bourdieu, P. (1984). *Distinction.* Cambridge, Mass.: Harvard University Press.

Brumberg, J. J. (2000). *Fasting Girls.* New York: Vintage Books.

Burstein, N. (2001). Shallow Hal. *The Harvard Crimson.* Retrieved August 30, 2014, from http://www.thecrimson.com/article/2001/11/9/shallow-hal-shallow-hal-the-new/.

Cahnman, W. J. (1968). The Stigma of Obesity. *The Sociological Quarterly*, 9, 283–299.

Cantarella, E. (1992). *Bisexuality in the Ancient World.* New Haven: Yale University Press.

Castells, M. (1996). *The Rise of the Network Society.* Malden, Mass.: Blackwell Publishers.

Catullus, G. & Lee, G. (1991). *The Poems of Catullus.* Oxford: Oxford University Press.

Cohen, S. (1972). *Folk Devils and Moral Panics.* London: MacGibbon and Kee.

Crossley, N. (2013). Habit and Habitus. *Body & Society*, 19, 136–161.

ExtremeFeeding (2012a). Force Feeding with the Tube: Advanced Techniques. Retrieved September 5, 2014, from http://extremefeeding.com/index.php/en/fatteners/item/210-force-feeding-with-the-tube-advanced-techniques.

DOI: 10.1057/9781137470461.0005

ExtremeFeeding (2012b). Immobile. Retrieved September 5, 2014, from http://extremefeeding.com/index.php/en/poems-admirations/item/164-immobile.

Featherstone, M. (2000). *Body Modification*. London: Sage.

Feed [Motion picture]. (2005). Australia: All At Once.

Foucault, M. (1973). *The Birth of the Clinic*. New York: Pantheon Books.

Foucault, M. (1977). *Discipline and Punish*. New York: Pantheon Books.

Foucault, M. (1985). *The Use of Pleasure*. New York: Pantheon Books.

Gamman, L. & Makinen, M. (1995). *Female Fetishism*. Washington Square, NY: New York University Press.

Germov, J. & Williams, L. (1999). *A Sociology of Food and Nutrition*. South Melbourne, Vic.: Oxford University Press.

Giddens, A. (1991). *Modernity and Self-Identity*. Stanford, CA: Stanford University Press.

Gies, L. (2008). How Material Are Cyberbodies? Broadband Internet and Embodied Subjectivity. *Crime, Media, Culture*, 4, 311–330.

Giovanelli, D. & Peluso, N. M. (2006) Feederism: A New Sexual Pleasure and Subculture. In Seidman, Fischer, & Meeks (Eds.) *Handbook of the New Sexuality Studies*. New York: Routledge.

Goffman, E. (1959). *The Presentation of Self in Everyday Life*. Anchor Books: London.

Goffman, E. (1963). *Stigma: Notes on the Management of Spoiled Identity*. Englewood Hills, NJ: Prentice-Hall.

Goffman, E. (1974). *Frame Analysis*. New York: Harper & Row.

Graham, M (2005). Chaos. In Kulick, D. & Meneley, A. (Eds.) *Fat: The Anthropology of an Obsession*. New York: Jeremy P Tarcher.

Hakim, C. (2015). the Male Sexual Deficit: A Social Fact of the 21st Century. *International Sociology*, 30, 314–335.

Hall, W., Carter, A., & Forlini, C. (2015). The Brain Disease Model of Addiction: Is It Supported by the Evidence and Has It Delivered on Its Promises? *The Lancet Psychiatry*, 2, 105–110.

Handberg, C., Thorne, S., Midtgaard, J., Vinther Nielsen, C., & Lomborg, K. (2014). Revisiting Symbolic Interactionism as a Theoretical Framework beyond the Grounded Theory Tradition. *Qualitative Health Research*. London: Sage.

Haworth, A. (2011). Forced to be Fat. *Marie Clare*. Retrieved May 15, 2015, from http://www.marieclaire.com/politics/news/a3513/forcefeeding-in-mauritania/.

Hester, J. (2009). Feast of Burden. *Bitch*, 44, 37–53.

DOI: 10.1057/9781137470461.0005

Jack Sprat (1639/2015). *Roud Folk Song Index*. Vaughan Williams Memorial Library. Retrieved January 23, 2015, from http://www.vwml.org/record/RoudFS/S299995.

Jutel, A. (2005). Weighing Health: The Moral Burden of Obesity. *Social Semiotics, 15*, 113–125.

Kaplowitz, P. B. (2008). Link between Body Fat and the Timing of Puberty. *Pediatrics, 121*, 208–217.

Kendler, K. S., Chen, X., Dick, D., Maes, H., Gillespie, N., Neale, M. C., & Riley, B. (2012). Recent Advances in the Genetic Epidemiology and Molecular Genetics of Substance Use Disorders. *Nature Neuroscience, 15*, 181–189.

Kipnis, L. (1996). *Bound and Gagged*. New York: Grove Press.

Kulick, D. & Meneley, A. (2005). *Fat*. New York: Penguin.

LaFraniere, S. (2007, July 4). Nouakchott Journal: In Mauritania, Seeking to End and Overfed Ideal. *New York Times*. Retrieved May 12, 2015, from http://www.nytimes.com/2007/07/04/world/africa/04mauritania.html?pagewanted=all&_r=0.

Martin, R. (2010). Fat Girls and Feeders. *Womanist Musings*. Retrieved August 30, 2014, from http://www.womanist-musings.com/2010/11/fat-girls-and-feeders.html.

Monaghan, L. F. (2005) Big Handsome Men, Bears and Others: Virtual Constructions of "Fat Male Embodiment". *Body & Society, 11*, 81–111.

Morahan-Martin, J. (2000) *Cyber Psychology & Behavior, 3*(5), October: 683–691. http://online.liebertpub.com/doi/abs/10.1089/10949310050191683.

Moore, A. (2010, November 29). Feed Me Now: Women Who Love Being Fat. *The Daily Telegraph*. Retrieved August 31, 2014, from http://www.telegraph.co.uk/women/sex/8155024/Feed-me-now-women-who-love-being-fat.html.

Murray, S. (2004). Locating Aesthetics: Sexing the Fat Woman. *Social Semiotics, 14*, 238–247.

Murray, S. (2008). *The Fat Female Body*. New York: Palgrave Macmillan.

O'Brien, J. (2011). Spoiled Group Identities and Backstage Work: A Theory of Stigma Management Rehearsals. *Social Psychology Quarterly, 74*, 291–309.

Orbach, S. (1978). *Fat Is a Feminist Issue*. New York: Paddington Press.

Pigs Be Pigs (2008). *A Fantastic Tale of Force Feeding and Massive Weight Gain*. Retrieved January 23, 2015, from http://willixartist.deviantart.com/art/quot-Pigs-Be-Pigs-quot-91932752.

DOI: 10.1057/9781137470461.0005

Pigs Is Pigs (1937/2015). Retrieved January 23, 2015, from https://www.youtube.com/watch?v=ulFqjU1KQVU.

Probyn, E. (2000). *Carnal Appetites*. London: Routledge.

Prohaska, A. (2013). Feederism: Transgressive Behavior or Same Old Patriarchal Sex? *International Journal of Social Science Studies*, 1, 104–112.

Prohaska, A. (2014). Help Me Get Fat! Feederism as Communal Deviance on the Internet. *Deviant Behavior*, 35, 263–274.

Pyle, N. and Loewy, M. (2009). Double Stigma: Fat Men and Their Male Admirers. In Rothblum, E. & Solovay, S. (Eds.) *The Fat Studies Reader*. New York: NYU Press.

Really (2014). Fat Girls and Feeders. Retrieved August 30, 2014, from http://really.uktv.co.uk/fat-girls-and-feeders/article/fat-girls-and-feeders/.

Rettie, R. (2009). Mobile Phone Communication: Extending Goffman to Mediated Interaction. *Sociology*, 43, 421–438.

Rosenberg, K. P. & Feder, L. C. (2014). *Behavioral Addictions*. San Diego: Academic Press.

Rosenberg, K. P., O'Connor, S., & Carnes, P. (2014). Sex Addiction: An Overview. In Paul, K. P. & Feder, L. C. (Eds.) *Behavioral Addictions*. San Diego: Academic Press.

Saugy, A. (2013). What's wrong with Fat? Oxford University Press. Oxford.

Sedgwick, E. (1990). *Epistemology of the Closet*. Berkeley: University of California Press.

Shilling, C. (2003). *The Body and Social Theory*. London: Sage Publications.

Simpson, D. (2014). Retrieved August 20, 2014, from http://www.officialdonnasimpson.com/index.html. [This site is no longer active].

Tenderlovingcares, (ed.) (2015). HORNGY, Issue 1. Retrieved February 20, 2015, from http://www.tlc-horngry.com/download-magazine/.

Terry, L. L. (2007). Food, Feeding, and Female Sexual Arousal. Unpublished master's thesis for master's degree, University of Lethbridge, Alberta, Canada. Retrieved August 31, 2014, from https://www.uleth.ca/dspace/bitstream/handle/10133/2510/terry,%20lesley.pdf?sequence=1.

Terry, L. L., Suschinsky, K. D., Lalumiere, M. L., & Vasey, P. L. (2012). Feederism: An Exaggeration of a Normative Mate Selection Preference? *Archives of Sexual Behavior*, 41, 249–260.

DOI: 10.1057/9781137470461.0005

Terry, L. L., & Vasey, P. L. (2011). Feederism in a Woman. *Archives of Sexual Behavior, 40*, 639–645.

Thege, B. K., Colman, I., el-Guedbaly, N., Hodgins, D. C., Patten, S. B., Schopflocher, D., Wolfe, J., & Wild, T. C. (2015). Social Judgments of Behavioral versus Substance-Related Addictions: A Population-Based Study. Addictive Behaviors, *42*, 24–31.

Thompson, C. S. (2014). Body Image in Mauritania: Bigger in Better. *Utah Historical Review, Volume IV*. Retrieved May 12, 2015, from http://epubs.utah.edu/index.php/historia/article/viewFile/1194/982.

Tischner, I (2013). *Fat Lives: A Feminist Psychological Exploration*. London: Routledge.

Walby, S. (1990). *Theorizing Patriarchy*. London: Blackwell Publishers.

Walter, N. (2010). *Living Dolls: The Return of Sexism*. London: Virago Press.

Wood, G. P. and E. H. Rudduck (1923). *Vitalogy or Encyclopedia of House and Home*. Chicago, Ill.: Vitalogy Association.

Yau, Y. H. C., Gottlieb, C. D., Krasna, L. C., & Potenza, M. N. (2014). Food Addiction: Evidence, Evaluation, and Treatment. In Paul, K. P. & Feder, L. C. (Eds.) *Behavioral Addictions*. San Diego: Academic Press.

DOI: 10.1057/9781137470461.0005

2
Personal Stories and Feederism Fiction

Abstract: *This chapter presents new data on feederism and offers a thematic analysis of semi-structured interviews with 23 participants who currently practice feederism. These data also include three romantic couples who were interviewed as couples, which presents a novel insight into the feederism experience. In addition to interviews, there is also a thematic analysis of five pieces of feederism fiction, which explores the more extreme end of feederism fantasy. Three super themes emerge from the analyses: early interest in fat (from early childhood in most cases); agency (showing a clear desire to reject feederism as coercive); and fantasy (highlighting extreme feederism practices as rare and fantasy-based rather than the norm).*

Charles, Kathy and Michael Palkowski. *Feederism: Eating, Weight Gain, and Sexual Pleasure.* Basingstoke: Palgrave Macmillan, 2015. DOI: 10.1057/9781137470461.0006.

 DOI: 10.1057/9781137470461.0006

Introduction

This chapter presents new findings from 23 interviews and an analysis of feederism fiction. The aim of the research was to address the gaps in existing literature on feederism, explore some of the assumptions linked to feederism, and to generate data that helps to develop new theory and practice centred on feederism. Some of the weaknesses in previous feederism research include a lack of diversity in participants, small numbers of participants, and a focus on extreme forms of feederism such as immobility. Most of the assumptions about feederism have tended to focus on patriarchal power dynamics, an absence of choice in female feedees, and potential psychopathology in the form of paraphilia such as masochism.

After gaining ethical approval from Edinburgh Napier University, participants for this research were recruited online. This was initially done by the first author writing a blog post about the project on her own blog and then tweeting this post several times. The authors also contacted one participant directly (Ruben) after visiting his website, extremefeeding.com. Ruben added the blog link to his site and that led to the first participant. Ruben participated in the research himself several months later. Eventually participants began to promote the research themselves on Tumblr and Twitter once they knew it was legitimate and had enjoyed taking part. Another participant (Gabriela) also promoted the research on her website and in her feederism magazine *HORNGRY*. This led to greatly increased interest, and unfortunately many participants were turned away as the project came to an end.

Once participants understood the nature of the research and completed a consent form, they were invited to take part in a real-time online interview using Skype. The date and time of the interview was negotiated by e-mail. To protect participants' privacy (and to allow telephone numbers to be called if necessary) interviews were conducted using voice only, rather than video. Each interview used a semi-structured interview schedule containing 12 questions (see below), and the duration of the interviews varied from 25 minutes to more than two hours. Some participants did not feel comfortable taking part in a real-time interview, so they provided typed responses to the questions and returned them by e-mail. Interview transcripts and typed responses were analysed using thematic analysis, and this is described further in the sections below.

DOI: 10.1057/9781137470461.0006

The role of the researcher was never hidden from participants in this study. Nobody was approached in the guise of fellow feeder or feedee, and the researchers did not establish fake profiles on feederism websites or pretend to be part of the feederism community. Researchers, journalists, and others setting up fake profiles and attempting to obtain information was cited as a major frustration from participants. Distrust of academics and journalists seems to be an issue, with a feeling in the community that they have been poorly represented by a false, one-dimensional narrative. All the participants in this study indicated that the mainstream portrayal of feederism was wrong, with several saying they were taking part as a way to rectify this disparity.

Interview schedule

Could you tell me what the term feederism means to you?

What terminology from feederism do you identify with?

Can you engage in feederism by yourself, or is it necessary to have another person involved?

When did you first start to feel that weight gain or feeding others was sexy?

Can you recall your first erotic experience with weight gain or a large body?

Can you remember when you first started to engage in eating (or feeding others) deliberately for weigh gain?

Could you tell me about meal times, do you eat a lot in one big meal time? Or do you eat frequently through the day? Can you remember what your eating patterns were like as a child?

Is there a sensory pleasure from eating (or preparing) food, such as the taste or the smell of it, or is food merely a means to an end? Are you more concerned with weight gain than with the experience of food itself?

Do other people who you know (friends, family, colleagues) know that you are involved in feederism?

If you have encountered mainstream documentaries on feederism, do you feel like they are representative of your own eating (or feeding) behaviour(s)?

Are you aware of force-feeding, tube-feeding, funnel-feeding, and the use of other equipment in feederism? If so, have you ever taken part in these things, and how do you feel about them?

DOI: 10.1057/9781137470461.0006

How do you feel about feeding to immobility in either a literal or fantasy context?

Participants

Twenty-three participants (12 males, 11 females) took part in the research. Sixteen (eight male, eight female) gave interviews while seven (four male, three female) provided written responses. The age, sexuality, and educational background of participants was not recorded, and this is discussed further in the limitations section of Chapter 3.

Stories

This chapter also presents an analysis of five pieces of feederism fiction from the *Dimensions Magazine* website (*Dimensions*, 2015). This sociological analysis uses the work of Lewis (2011), which sees storytelling as a way of understanding the lived world and understanding our own identity and the identity of others.

The remainder of the chapter is divided into three sections. The first section details the key themes and analysis that emerged from respondents who typed their responses to the interview questions. This is followed by an analysis of the themes that emerged from real-time semi-structured interviews, followed by an overview of the common themes across all participants. The second section details analysis of feederism fiction from *Dimensions Magazine*, with the final section providing a summary conclusion.

Section 1

Part 1 – Written responses

Seven participants chose to take part in this research by providing typed answers rather than being interviewed. Some participants felt shy about being interviewed and were concerned that they might be overheard by friends or family members. Others preferred to write their answers so that they could think about their responses a little more or because English was

DOI: 10.1057/9781137470461.0006

not their first language. Participants who took part in this way answered the same questions as those who were interviewed. Five themes emerged in the analysis of written responses: childhood feelings and experiences with fat; the labelling of feederism; secrecy in feederism; attitudes towards extreme behaviours; and the public narrative of feederism. The participants were Mina, Joshua, JD, Roger, Diane, Jess, and Herbert.

Childhood feelings and experiences with fat (including first sexual feelings)

The first theme centres on two kinds of experience and feeling, which tend to overlap. The first was fantasizing about other people gaining weight, and the second was thinking sexually about gaining weight themselves.

Pillows

Pillows are a recurring object in the transcripts when considering early weight gain experiences. Mina notes that she could trace her feedist roots back to the age of three years old. She would stuff pillows underneath her clothing to perform a fat body. These sentiments are described almost word for word by Joshua who noted, "When I was a child I remember me playing with some pillows under my clothes trying to be fat." Pretending and playing out the role of the fat body would persist throughout her childhood but with a particular fascination on her stomach and on growing her body. Performing the fat body meant being able to experiment with fantasized growth, which would also change the self. Herbert similarly discussed the idea of pillows, but in a slightly different way. He noted, "I have always had a fascination with fat people and weight gain since I was very young. As early as three I can remember being upset because my mother had lost weight from an illness and 'my nice pillow' was gone from her lap." Interestingly in this instance the pillow is no longer there and weight has been lost. The performative potential of the pillow for young children in being fat seems to be pertinent. Herbert in his written response noted, "I used to pretend that my imaginary friends would gain weight for whatever reason." Externalized weight gain is a performative aspect here.

Fat representations

Media depictions of fat, typically looking at weight gain as a disorder that needs rectifying, is very memorable for the written participants.

DOI: 10.1057/9781137470461.0006

There were specific references to magazine articles and cartoons where elaborate fat is portrayed, often for comic effect. Remembering larger characters on television was a recurring theme in the sample. Herbert noted the following in his responses, "I also remember reading my mother's women's magazines and the articles in them about 'My problem and how I solved it" type subjects where the women's 'problem" was that they gained a lot of weight and then how they lost it. Those articles usually described the process of how they got fat in great detail, and I liked to read them."

Cartoons also provided a representation of fat intrigue as Mina was fixated by characters in television shows that became fat. Mina notes for example, "Later in childhood I had a fascination with my belly, and certain cartoons where a character got fat intrigued me (but I had no clue why)." These characters typically transformed to such an extent that they were not recognizable in their different forms; it was a total transformation from one person to another. These feelings and thoughts did not fully make sense until Mina became aware of and part of the active feederism community, where she recognized her feelings of fat admiration and her love of gaining weight.

Joshua also discussed the ways in which celebrities who had gained weight in gossip magazines were appealing and also how larger girls were seen as more attractive: "When I was 9 y.o. I really liked to see in some magazines pictures of famous people who gained weight. I also liked the girls that gained weight at school."

JD believes that he first had thoughts of feederism at 12 years old, which was brought about by a fascination with larger breasts. This occurred after seeing a picture in the Guinness Book of World Records (GBWR) of a woman with very large natural breasts (a category that remains in the publication (GBWR, 2015) and has been held by the same woman since 1999). The blueberry expansion scene of Violet Beauregard in the movie *Willy Wonka and the Chocolate Factory* is also isolated as an example that excited JD. He goes on to elaborate that he watched this scene on repeat and was "incredibly fascinated." There is a sense of wonderment in seeing fat bodies displayed as oddities, particularly something that could be rewarded, or be the result of something gone wrong.

Roger notes that at the beginning of his adolescence, he watched a particular episode of the cartoon "Totally Spies," which was called "Passion Patties," in which one of the female protagonists gets hooked on addictive and fattening foods. The episode interested him, but he did

DOI: 10.1057/9781137470461.0006

not fully comprehend why this was. He felt aroused, and the episode stuck with him to such a degree that he credits the episode with him discovering feederism online. He was able to learn about the fetish and to understand that there were like-minded people. He notes "This story seems to be quite common as far as I've read on feederism discussion boards." Roger remembers that his first sexual experience was at the age of 16 with a "thin girl," which was not arousing to him. He remarks that he had a relationship with a girl at the age of 17 who was a gainer, an experience he remembers as arousing as it linked with his erotic experiences of early life, particularly the cartoon he remembered so fondly.

Mina recognized that her first erotic experience was with her own body, in feeling different fat parts of herself: "I've never been a small person; I've always been fat. Touching my body felt good, right even. It's the same even now. Every little touch, whether it's from someone else or from myself, it feels natural."

Labelling

For JD, feederism is "a fetish of erotically controlling another person's or your own eating" and is associated with overeating with the intention of fattening up a participant. This is contrasted with Mina, who remarks that feederism is a fetish which is "comprised of [*sic*] people who find pleasure in gaining weight, watching someone else gain weight or both." Mina prefers using the term feedism because for her it is more neutral and does not imply a relational dynamic of control. Mina believes that there is a misconception that the feeder is the beneficiary of all the pleasure whilst the feedee is an unwilling participant in the dynamic. Feedism is used to differentiate and move away from the stereotype. Roger remarks that feederism is also a subculture and an identity. It is not simply about the act of being a feeder or a feedee, it is about partaking in a larger "culture of acceptance" which is "derived from the taboo of their fetish." This sense of cultural cohesiveness is due to the marginalization and perceived deviancy of the act but also in the sense of acceptance that results in embracing a deviant identity. Roger regards this as a "libertarian, don't-tell-me-what-to-do bent." This therefore places significant agency on the individual in realizing his or her own sexuality and using the community as a way to facilitate this. This is reiterated by Diane who described feederism as an act of rebellion and freedom of expression: "Feederism to me is an act of rebellion. Rebelling against the norm,

DOI: 10.1057/9781137470461.0006

rebelling against societies [*sic*] beauty standards, feederism is a way for me to be me." It allows her to be a "fatter version of myself with each gain" and therefore showcases a type of transformation of the self.

Jess described feederism as a dynamic between a feedee, who has an attraction to overeating intentionally to gain weight, and a feeder, who has an interest in helping the feedee gain weight by encouraging them to overeat or actually by feeding them through purchasing or preparing food for them.

The ways participants defined feederism more broadly affected the ways they chose to sub-label their identities within the feederism subculture. JD, for example, notes the fluidity of labels and the sexual performances that are associated with feederism. He notes that he used to be a feedee, then a feeder, and now recognizes himself as a mutual gainer. This change in labelling shows a tendency that is common within our sample to move between different roles either in a literal context or within a fantasy world. Mina notes that she is a feedee, but that she has "mutual gaining tendencies." This tendency to take part in a mutual gaining relationship is dependent entirely on her partner. If her partner is not interested in gaining weight, then she is simply a "feedee" but she can "play both roles." She notes that regardless of her partner, she retains her "feedee side." Her sexual default setting is gaining weight, and as such it can "definitely be a solo activity." Mina prefers being with a partner to share her fetish, but this is simply a preference rather than a requirement. Jess similarly has mutual gaining tendencies and enjoys watching other people overeat. She considers herself a feedee and a mutual gainer, using both terms to incorporate how she likes watching other people gain. Autoerotic feeding for Jess is viewed as being impossible because of the social stigma of being fat. She requires the support and encouragement of a feeder, but interestingly she only requires an online feeder and does not want to actively become involved with a feeder in person. It is almost as though permission is required to keep eating.

In contrast, Diane considers herself strictly a feedee or a gainer, but this feedee role is very much an assertive role. Since Diane views feederism as an act of rebellion and an act of disavowing beauty standards, the agency in gaining weight and transforming her body is her own. Diane has engaged in autoerotic forms of feederism and describes purposely gaining 40 lbs. to see if her partner would notice: "Prior to learning that my partner (now husband) was a feeder, I had purposefully put on 40 pounds to see if he would notice, and he had. I explained to him that I enjoy gaining weight

DOI: 10.1057/9781137470461.0006

for sexual pleasure. That is when I learned he is a feeder/encourager." Autoerotic feeding was used as a way of testing the waters and to see if her partner would be interested in helping her gain weight.

Roger regards himself as an encourager because he has never done any feeding himself but again insists that he "probably would engage in feeding with a willing partner and derive sexual pleasure from it." He discredits the idea of an autoerotic form of feeding because he considers himself an "encourager" which requires another person as part of the relationship. JD notes that autoerotic forms of feederism are part of a larger community because often gaining weight is encouraged on blogs and forums. Being alone has different connotations and significance for JD because even if you prefer being by yourself, you can post pictures of your progress on sites like Tumblr, and you can find your own "set of fans based on gender/weight/interest" as a result. Like Jess, some kind of external encouragement or appreciation is necessary.

An interesting labelling conflict was uncovered in Herbert's written response. He noted the following: "Part of it was the fact that I wanted to be a physician, and being fat and getting fatter was strictly seen as unhealthy. I struggled with those questions all through medical school as well. How could I like something which was unhealthy? How could I encourage someone to make themselves unhealthier? It took me a long time to resolve those issues. As time passed, I learned that being fat is not necessarily unhealthy. I learned about the HAES (health at every size) movement. I also started to realize that people who engaged in this fetish were well aware of the risks it posed and still chose to engage in it anyway."

Being in medical school meant that Herbert was exposed to a specific frame about fat, which encouraged a certain understanding of fat. To be large meant to be unhealthy, and it was a taken-for-granted assumption that it resulted in significant difficulties for Herbert in dealing with his own fetish. He eventually realized that people within the community tend to know the risks involved in gaining weight and that fat in-of-itself is not typically associated with unhealthy bodies. A significant labelling conflict, or dissonance, arose because two different aspects of Herbert's life appeared incompatible. These conflicts meant that Herbert merely "lurked" online on feederism websites and forums for 13 years, instead of actively participating. It also affected the types of women that he felt like he could date: "There were other issues that needed to be resolved before I felt like I could date (a big one being some severe bullying I went

DOI: 10.1057/9781137470461.0006

through as a child in 7th grade in school), so from 1995 to 2008 I mainly 'lurked' on the feederism web sites...reading them but not actively participating."

Herbert eventually became more active in 2009, when he was more comfortable being a medical doctor and having a weight gain fetish. It also meant he could clear up medical misconceptions that were on these sites. He also felt like he had an insider status as a doctor: "In 2009 I joined Fantasy Feeder and started chatting. By then I was comfortable with being a physician with a weight gain fetish and I saw lots of medical misconceptions that people on the fetish sites had and I figured that I could help clear them up. I was "one of them" so they might be more willing to listen to me."

Secrecy

Another notable theme that emerged from the data is the novel ways in which secrecy was represented. Roger notes that due to the stigma associated with feederism he has only revealed it to a few friends who he feels would understand and keep it a secret. He goes on to remark, "Keeping my sexuality hidden is quite pressuring, so that is why I have chosen to talk about it to some friends." Similarly JD talks about secrecy by stating that he does not share it with anyone in his family or with any friends. Even those closest to him are unaware of his fetish: "Out of 25 past partners, I have felt comfortable to share with only 3." He explains that this is because of a bad reaction he got from a previous partner.

Roger refers to this process as an "outing" and this sense of "outing oneself" is significant, as it suggests that feederism is not just a sexual fetish that fits within a preconceived sexual discourse, but rather is its own unique form. Mina notes that she has a lot of friends in the online feederism community and a few offline friends as well, but that she does not consider it a vital piece of information to disclose to other people. She states that the sex lives of her colleagues, acquaintances and family are none of her business and therefore her sexual habits and desires are equally none of theirs. This suggests a spectrum, where for some people, outing is a significant process of making themselves feel comfortable with who they are as people since feederism is such a major part of their identity, but for others "outing" themselves is not as significant. This differentiation may be a reflection of how immersed an individual is in online communities as being visible already within a group that already

DOI: 10.1057/9781137470461.0006

understands, reinforces and encourages your self-identity makes coming out less significant offline.

Herbert expressed a general comment about the feederism community, "not very many feederists tell their friends and family about the fetish. Being fat and gaining weight are not seen as positive things and so the fetish is very poorly understood. Most families and friends would have a negative reaction." However he also noted that he has a close relationship with his mother, who he has told about it, and "she was very non-judgmental so I was able to tell her about feederism and my interest in it. I have also been able to tell my brother and his wife about it as well. They have all been accepting, though my brother does find the idea a little odd." The feeling of secrecy is linked to how poorly we understand fat fetishism and how we negatively discuss it more generally.

Extreme

Force-feeding and the use of equipment such as funnels and tubes were viewed by a number of the participants to be practically unsuitable to their desires or particular fetish outside of a fantasy. Mina, for example, states that she has not taken part in force-feeding or used any forms of equipment and regards tube-feeding in particular as quite dangerous. She believes that she would be open to the idea of engaging in forced and more coercive forms of gaining if this was done in a mutually consensual way whereby the coercion was part of an act. She states that similar to forms of BDSM, there should be a safe word or signal for the passive partner to indicate that they are no longer consenting. This is a situation which is shared by Roger, who believes that clear-cut boundaries and consent are vital. JD, in contrast, considers it in a more pragmatic way, and believes they are not effective. He states, "Even a 300lbs woman can only hold a relatively small amount of liquid."

In other cases, tube-feeding was viewed as something that could be achieved with willing partners but only in the right circumstances. Herbert writes, "I am aware of all of those feeding modalities. In the right context they can be fun. If I had a partner that wanted to do some of those things I would probably try them. But only with a willing partner."

Immobility was also viewed as impractical, but was often fantasized about. Roger notes that whilst he respects other people choosing to feed to immobility, he does not have a preference for very large women. In a fantasy, there are no health risks, and so its portrayal is regarded as

DOI: 10.1057/9781137470461.0006

less problematic. Mina similarly differentiates fantasies from real life, in that immobility is only practical and possible in the imaginary. Getting larger would mean a loss of individuality for Mina, as she describes it as "not being able to move around and being able to go out and do various things." Similarly JD comments: "The thought of becoming immobile or having an immobile partner is erotic but not realistic. It is strictly a fantasy." Herbert notes, "Immobility is a fun fantasy, but it's just that. A fantasy. It's just not practical. Being a physician I am fully aware of the work that it takes for someone to care for someone else who is completely immobile and completely dependent on someone to do everything for them."

There was also specific weight limits that were imposed arbitrarily on gaining that detracted from the possibility of having literal immobility. Joshua, for example, writes, "it´s just a fantasy. i have fantasies about getting so fat i cant move and also i have fantasies about gettting a girl inmobile. in real life i wouldnt like to get fatter than around 250 pounds. and also i wont like that my girlfriend got immobile. Around 400 pounds would be perfect [*sic*]". Arbitrary weight limits allowed for a practical self and an extreme fantasized self to coexist.

Public narrative

The public narrative of feederism was viewed universally as negative and unrepresentative of the participants' lived experiences. The representation of feederism is seen as extreme and inconsistent with the community. All of the written responses conveyed this. Mina states that documentaries, talk show specials, movies and so on are terrible portrayals of feederism. "They seem to take the most extreme of us and paint us all with that brush! Some of these people make me ashamed to have this fetish. We are NOT the monsters we are made out to be. The vast majority of us are not victims or abusers. We are not all this extreme about weight gain." Similarly Herbert writes, "They paint a picture of feederists as being mentally ill or totally manipulative. Feeders are all seen as sexual predators taking advantage of poor fat women, making them too fat to move and then leaving them helpless and moving on to their next victim. It makes for great television, but totally paints an unrealistic view of the fetish."

JD regards the mainstream portrayal of feederism to be "very negative and sensational." This is because, according to JD, an obese woman

DOI: 10.1057/9781137470461.0006

is typically being dominated by a man, with the woman having no control or say over the situation. He goes on to say: "The overwhelming majority of feeding is consensual. There is even peer pressure for those to shout down or delete content that is not consensual in the Feederism community." Roger goes on to discuss the ways in which he believes documentary makers artificially create the notion that feederism is somehow alien, disgusting, weird or contemptible. The sensationalized aspect means that informative and detailed content is brushed aside, often presenting the subculture in an unsympathetic light. Roger says, "The shock value of the film is seen as more important than the informative content and there is little to no empathy or sympathy."

Roger is aware of the health frame and discusses the ways in which various public institutions come together to actively "shun or discourage" the fetish. Society has a preference for thin bodies, which, combined with the "obesity epidemic," means that feederism is viewed in a very negative light. Roger says that this is a major motivating factor for his involvement in this project: "This is one of the reasons I am participating in this study: I can't change my sexuality and would prefer not to be shunned for it."

Summary of written responses

The findings from the typed responses identify many issues relating to early life experiences, the labelling of feederism, secrecy, and attitudes to extreme activities. The next section explores the responses of interviewees who were interviewed in real time, and the similarities between the two groups are clear. Themes and examples identified in written responses are repeated in the interviews along with additional experiences and perspectives.

Section 1

Part 2 – Semi-structured interviews

Ten individual participants (five male, five female) were interviewed online in real time using Skype. One participant (Grayson) was interviewed

DOI: 10.1057/9781137470461.0006

twice. A further six individuals were interviewed as romantic couples (two male-female couples online using Skype and one male-female couple face-to-face at Edinburgh Napier University). Couples have not been interviewed together in feederism research before, so they are presented as a separate group here to reflect the unique interview dynamic. Each interview in this section tells a different feederism story, and each one is discussed separately with its own set of themes. Similarities inevitably emerge, and a bigger picture summary is presented at the end of the section.

Ruben

Ruben is the owner and creator of a website called extremefeeding.com. It is a long-established site created in 1999 and was previously called Ruben's Feeder. Ruben now has a Facebook page, Twitter account, Tumblr blog, and uploads YouTube videos all dedicated to feederism. Ruben's output is somewhat unique, as it is bilingual, with content in both English and German. His site has come under some criticism from Prohaska (2014), who highlights one of Ruben's projects dedicated to feeding and photographing a woman as she gained weight (he called her his "fattening cow"). Nevertheless, Ruben's output has become progressively diverse (poems, fiction, podcasts, artwork), and he also publicizes the work of others. Aspects of Ruben's site attempt to have an educative function much like his YouTube videos. He is keen to describe feederism to the outside world and to reinforce the consensual nature of it. The first page of his site requires users to confirm they are aged over 18 and says, "the theme of this site is to consentually [*sic*] feed and fatten up people. It is about fat, fattening and the people that love both. If this is your thing, you'll find a lot of fun stuff in here." Undoubtedly most of the content is highly sexualized, and some of the fantasy components describe coercive situations, but these alternate between males and females taking the coercive role. Most of the content is far from the mainstream idea of feederism being about coercive males fattening females. One of the most recent fantasy stories posted by Ruben involves a male feedee meeting a slim woman with a medical degree who specializes in gastroenterology and can help him get fatter quicker by taking on the excess weight of another man (ExtremeFeeding, 2014). This does not fit the common feederism narrative, even though there are some examples of that narrative on the site. Ruben himself also identifies as both a feeder and a feedee (ExtremeFeeding, 2015).

DOI: 10.1057/9781137470461.0006

Meaning of feederism and early experiences

When Ruben was interviewed for the current research, he requested that his responses use the name Ruben rather than a pseudonym. Ruben described feederism as "a thing I got to know about myself... like homosexuality to a gay person." He says that it is "big in my life, important, and I love it." Just as his website suggests, he identified himself as feeder, feedee, and mutual gainer during the interview, and was comfortable with this flexibility, although he says he was strictly a feeder until four years ago. Ruben identified his interest in fat as dating back "as far as I can remember" and he says this kind of lifelong fascination is common among users of his site, claiming that 30 or 40 individual people had specifically told him the same thing. As with other participants in this research he talks of finding "chubby" girls attractive at school. He reports having felt, at age 13, that his fantasies about weight gain were "really, really dangerous" and that they might come true and get out of hand.

At age 19 or 20, Ruben began to write erotic stories about feederism and initially felt very fearful that they would be discovered. He describes doing this as a way to experiment with his sexual feelings and "reveal his desires". When he first decided to publish his stories on his website, he felt very scared and anticipated hate mail and even death threats. The positive feedback he received encouraged him to develop his site further, and he now sees it as a place where a number of people have finally come to understand their own desires. Ruben has assumed the role of a self-styled educator on the subject of feederism, and he feels very comfortable telling curious visitors to his site what feederism is and assigning identities to them (e.g. identifying them as a feedee or feeder). He is also proud of the meet-ups he has arranged in California so that people involved in feederism can see that other people look the same as them and are not "monsters." He suggests that this can help people feel more comfortable with their identities, and he conjectures that most anxiety around feederism is caused by the fear of how other people might judge it.

Two sides

At several points in his interview, Ruben presents a Manichaean perspective on thinking and behaviour. He describes himself as feeling like Dr. Jekyll and Mr. Hyde. He talks of uniting "the feeder and feedee within," a person having two parts: "conforming and giving in," and feedees needing to be "courageous" enough to admit they want to be forced to gain and accept their feederism. He appears keen on presenting the idea of

DOI: 10.1057/9781137470461.0006

internal conflict and this possibly reflects his own experience of moving from fearing his fantasies and being terrified of weight gain to being extremely public about his interests and claiming that he "inspire[s] men to gain." It may also reflect the obvious childhood conflict he experienced having overweight parents who constantly commented on him getting "as fat as us" and "not able to do anything" whilst maintaining their own weight.

Extreme side of feederism

When Ruben is asked about force-feeding and immobility, he admits an interest in both but feels that immobility is mostly a fantasy concept. He even suggests it may be a key fantasy script for those who are not able to gain weight in real life because they have jobs that require a certain image. He has considered equipment that he might design and build to make his life easier if he became immobile but he mostly confines it to a fantasy, commenting that "sexual energy can inflate ... fantasies to crazy proportions." Immobility has often featured in feederism documentaries, which have depicted apparently rare incidences of a feedee reaching immobility. Ruben dislikes these documentaries, believing them to stereotype the subculture and be biased and sad. He feels that the women in them are portrayed as sad victims when the reality of the female feedees he knows is that they are "strong women." He acknowledges that he has met male feeders who he feels "have no moral compass" and over feed women who just happen to enjoy eating rather than being feedees. Ruben finds this distasteful and not genuine feederism. He appears to make a clear distinction between some of the fantasies on his website and his real-life behaviour and experiences.

Promoting alternative views

Ruben's site has recently (24 December 2014) promoted an online magazine called *HORNGRY*. The magazine is designed for male feedees and female feeders. It provides a glossary of terms used in feederism, including an explanation of different vocabulary used by gay and straight feeders/feedees along with quite extensive information on what feederism is all about. It also includes interviews with female feeders (one with username 'I feed bears') and male feedees (the gainer of the month called 'one deadly sin') along with photographs, fiction stories and art work. The magazine has a very positive tone and does not have an agenda of coercion. It appears traditionally "feminine" in its styling

DOI: 10.1057/9781137470461.0006

(e.g. pastel shades and the use of flowers) with much of the content praising fat male bodies (e.g. "a love letter to stretch marks"). The designer of the magazine (Gabriela) is a psychology graduate who herself is keen to raise awareness of what feederism is and to counter the image portrayed by documentaries like *Fat Girls and Feeders* (discussed in the introduction). Gabriela was interviewed for this research and her contribution is discussed below. All of the contributors to *HORNGRY* appear to use a site called Grommr which claims to be "a social network... for gainers, bloaters, encouragers and admirers" (Grommr, 2015). This site organizes meet ups for members in cities in several different countries. Again, the message is positive rather than coercive or humiliating. In the "about" section of Grommr, there is an acknowledgement that many people involved in feederism developed the interest early life and had always felt drawn to larger bodies. The site attracts a lot of gay men, so a newer site called Feabie.com has been created for "the needs of the heterosexual feederism community" whilst also welcoming people of all orientations (Feabie, 2015).

Gabriela

Gabriela identifies as a female feeder, and she is the editor of *HORNGRY*. In *HORNGRY* the larger male body is the object of desire and it fits in with research focused on "handsome bears" (Monaghan, 2005). Gabriela was interviewed as a participant in this research, as her identity as a female feeder represents a rarely addressed group in feederism research. Gabriela also interviewed the authors for *HORNGRY* so that she could report on the progress of the research and encourage participation.

Labelling

Gabriela considers feederism to be an extension of her personality. To say it is a lifestyle is too cliché, and so she remarks, "I like to take care of people, I like to take care of a man and like cooking and feeding for him is just part of that." The female feeder role here is synonymous with the traditional female role of providing nourishment for the male in the home. Gabriela stated that weight gain does not have to be involved in the dynamic, as feeding is the main focus. Consequently the term feederism is not one that Gabriela likes to use because of the associations it has. Shying away from the term feederism is a recurring theme in some of the

DOI: 10.1057/9781137470461.0006

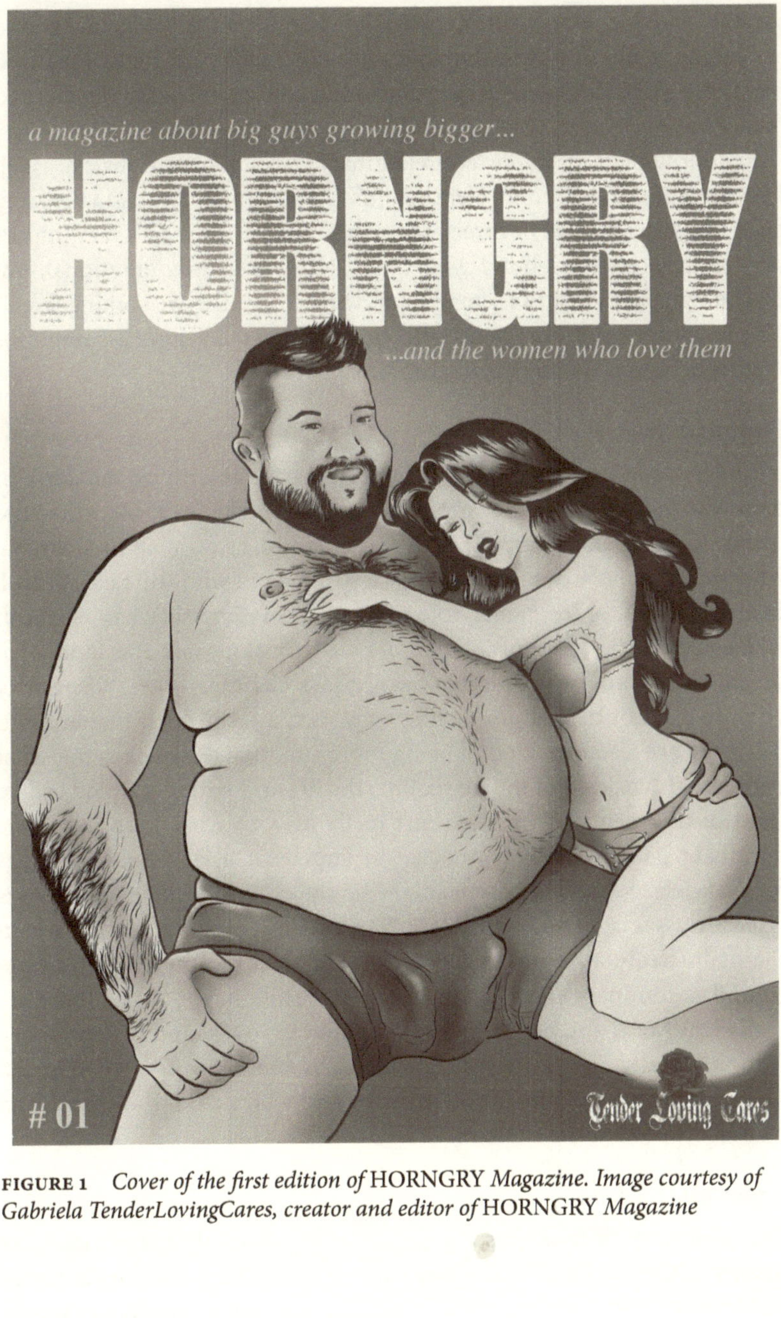

FIGURE 1 *Cover of the first edition of* HORNGRY *Magazine. Image courtesy of Gabriela TenderLovingCares, creator and editor of* HORNGRY *Magazine*

DOI: 10.1057/9781137470461.0006

sample. Moving away from negative labels means that judgements and assumptions about power dynamics are not made. Gabriela's preferred terms are gainer and encourager due to the connotations that feedee and feeder have.

Encouraging is an important relationship dynamic for Gabriela: "Well I've been lurking around websites for a long time. I've actually only encouraged about two or three men so far because for me it's very important to have a strong bond with them. Not necessarily emotional, but just being able to talk to them and knowing where they're coming from." This apparent emotional bond with encouraging challenges assumptions that feederism is mostly pornographic or coercive.

Dominant gainer

An interesting part of Gabriela's interview was describing the sorts of men who gain. Usually they are submissive and take on a role where the female is more dominant. This dynamic is not favourable to Gabriela, who prefers a more dominant gainer, a strong man who will take control. The dominant feedee/gainer role is another subtlety that has not been addressed in the literature, but it shows that alongside the fluidity of sexual roles comes the fluidity of power. As Gabriela notes, "Especially because a lot of men, I don't know why, but, a lot of men that are into being fed are also into kind of being more submissive, which is not what I am into. I like kind of the masculine; the big and strong guy and so like most of the men I see online don't really fit with what I am into." The dominant gainer role is connected to larger social and cultural issues for Gabriela. We asked why it might be the case that the gainer role is typically associated with humiliation and submissiveness, particularly in the mainstream accounts of feederism. Gabriela responded, "I have yet to find a dominant male German gainer. While in the States there are really loads of them, but they're really far away so it's kind of depressing. I think it really has to do with it being such a taboo in society to be fat. The people who are already submissive and who are kind of turned on by that it makes sense to them."

Importance of food

The sensuality of food was a key part of the arousal for Gabriela. The quality of the food and the presentation of it was important. It cannot be stated that food was simply about gaining calories or producing weight gain. Gabriela stated: "No, the food is very important for me. I just love

DOI: 10.1057/9781137470461.0006

to see a guy that really enjoys the food and likes to eat a lot because he loves it so much, not because he just wants to get big. I really love it so much. For example one of the hugest turn ons for me is when a guy like moans because he just likes the food, you know just like the way people do sometimes it's not a big thing, but for me it is." Contrary to a lot of our sample, it seemed that Gabriela was more interested in larger appetites than larger bodies. She noted when discussing a question she posted in her magazine: "I have this one question in there for Feeders – would you rather prefer someone big with a small appetite or a smaller guy that has a huge appetite and I'm definitely for the second, I just love to see a man eat a lot which is – the weight gain is amazingly hot, but it comes kind of second to the food and the pleasure."

Online presence

Gabriela was what others in the sample have termed a "lurker" in that she routinely visited fetish websites from an early age but only began to participate when older. She noted: "I've been actively on the websites and looking into and just reading weight gain fiction and stuff like that since I was about 13 – even 12, maybe. But I didn't have any contact with people until I'd say 17 or 18. But a lot more, recently, since I have to make a zine and cover and everything." A theme in our sample is that often people will peruse fetish sites and view the interactions taking place for a while before taking part. Immersion therefore is both active and passive when looking at interactions with fetish websites.

Extreme

Immobility and the more extreme aspects of feederism were viewed as unappealing due to the specific preference Gabriela has for her gainer: "I'm not into that [immobility] I don't know, my preferred body type would be kind of like what the gay community calls the muscle chub, which means like a big beefy strong man type of guy with a belly that's what I love most." The belly here is a fixated object, which can be focused on as a representation or indication of someone with a large, voracious appetite. It is combined with standardized masculine attributes, such as strength and power. The body is therefore a canvas for two distinct social messages. The first of these is a willingness to take control and have the means to do so, a type of hegemonic masculinity (Connell, 2006). The second is allowing yourself to be cared for and to be groomed within the domestic space, and to be provided for.

DOI: 10.1057/9781137470461.0006

Immobility and other forms of feederism, such as tube-feeding, are considered by Gabriela as indicative of one side of an extreme spectrum which has been unfairly painted as being representative of the entire fetish. She notes, "And it's very limited view of it. It's like there are extremes, even in this kink. I mean I won't lie there are people that participate in tube feeding which can be very dangerous, people that are into immobility and stuff like that. But it's like with BDSM there are extremes, but no kink wants to be represented by the most extreme edges of it instead of what most people practice, which is safe and consensual and pleasing to both."

Gabriela revealed a totally different area of feederism that was almost hidden in the academic literature. The female feeder role has a lot to say that challenges portrayals of feederism as being representative of patriarchal sexual dynamics (Prohaska, 2013) and has a lot to say about the huge diversity in body types, submissive versus dominant roles, and notions of extremity in the community.

Grayson

Grayson is the only participant in this research to have been interviewed twice. He was the first participant in the study and showed considerable interest in the research. Each interview lasted more than an hour, and Grayson also supplied several photographs of himself purporting to show a 70 lbs weight gain (he asked for these images not to be published). Grayson's first interview followed the semi-structured interview schedule, whilst the second interview explored specific themes in more detail. Significant themes in Grayson's interviews were humiliation and approach avoidance.

Early life and humiliation

Grayson described feederism as a fetish and a "turn on" but not something he chose. His first arousal connected to feederism happened when he was 12 years old, when a girl from school gained 30–40 lbs. while being away ill for a month. He had "always" liked larger bodies but was fascinated by the *rate* of weight gain in this case.

Grayson has tried to "get away" from feederism, but he keeps coming back to it. The humiliation aspect is exciting to him and he describes wanting gynecomastia (the benign growth of breast tissue in a male) so that his breasts become so large he cannot hide them and he is ridiculed.

DOI: 10.1057/9781137470461.0006

He specifically says that this would be "exciting" rather than something that would make him happy. He also fantasizes about being strapped to a chair and fed till he bursts. He claims to have hired a dominatrix before who has tied him to a chair and force-fed him cake and milk in an effort to act this out. He gets aroused by the idea that a woman would make fun of him for gaining weight and that she wouldn't like it.

Grayson is a user of the amateur pornography site Clips4Sale, and through this site he met someone who had gained weight and wanted to lose it. He emailed her and offered to eat her food for her. He claims to have gained 30 lbs. by eating whatever the woman told him to each day. He then orchestrated a situation where she blackmailed him if he didn't continue to gain weight.

Although Grayson enjoys humiliation he doesn't want his partner to be humiliated and is very clear that he doesn't want to humiliate women. He sometimes wants to dominate but feels he has no right to dominate so he dominates himself at times through autoerotic feeding. He then goes on to describe how much he would enjoy tube- or funnel-feeding, as he would have no choice but to consume and gain. The concept of no control is very stimulating to him, and there is possibly an approach/avoidance conflict with the concept of immobility. It excites Grayson, and he's attracted to it, yet he fears it. He is aroused by the morphing of the body and the exaggeration of the features. He is excited by someone having control over him. The health issues worry him to an extent, but not significantly. He is willing to embrace the danger of significant overeating because he thinks he could die anyway even if he takes care of himself. Robinson, Wilkowski, and Meier (2008) give an overview of approach avoidance in their study focusing on extraversion and neuroticism.

Feederism is a secret in Grayson's life, and he claims the interview for this research is the first time he has discussed feederism and his fantasies in such a way. He says that he's never told anyone what is inside him and who he is.

Grayson's attitude towards humiliation was explored further as it appeared to be a key factor in the blackmail dynamic he orchestrated and in his first interview. He described feeling embarrassed at age 12 because he had breasts. He found this embarrassment exciting and it has remained part of his sexuality since then. He described his life up until the age of 10 as being abusive, as his biological father was violent towards his mother and then his stepfather was also very violent towards the whole family.

DOI: 10.1057/9781137470461.0006

His stepfather left when he was 10 years old, and then Grayson had no father figure. He feels a resentment towards his mother for allowing there to be so much violence within the family when he was a child.

Loss of control

Grayson was interviewed a second time in order to fully explore some of the themes that emerged following his first interview (particularly humiliation, loss of control, and blackmail). Grayson had been in touch by e-mail between interviews to say that he had a new weight gain target, so this was the first thing that was explored in his second interview. Grayson was gaining weight through a new online relationship. He had been told by his female feeder to gain 25 lbs. (taking his weight to 325 lbs.) or face having personal information about himself posted on the internet. Grayson's concern about being exposed online was very real, yet he described his emotions on learning about his new weight target as "scared but at the same time it excites me." This links to the idea of an approach/avoidance conflict where he is simultaneously desiring and fearful of the same thing. To achieve this goal he described his recent food intake as "a lot of fast food. Pizza, Italian food, pastries, milkshakes, stuff like that." When asked if his feeder was interested in getting him immobile he replied "there is a possibility." In an effort to understand the blackmail dynamic, Grayson was asked to break down what would happen if he failed to comply with his online feeder. He described how embarrassing pictures of himself and his phone number would be linked to his real name so that they came up in Google searches. He was quite insistent that this could lead to his employer and friends finding out about his interests.

Grayson feels that feederism ("this fetish," as he calls it) has ruined his relationships with women because he can't share it with them. His inability to share it means that he retreats into his own fantasy world and seeks out online "mistresses." He feels that his real-life female partners don't understand that he wants to "live" feederism and not just do it occasionally. He feels it is a significant issue affecting his life. He says "it is everything I do now. It is an addiction," and later, "there has to be something... to totally obliterate it." Grayson's conflict with feederism couldn't be more obvious. He wants to be immersed in it and has set up a situation that forces him to be, yet he also dreads it and wants it out of his life. In no other participant does this conflict appear so starkly.

DOI: 10.1057/9781137470461.0006

Saskia, Gemma, Benny, Gavin

The interviews analysed above featuring Ruben, Gabriela, and Grayson are unique because of the professional interest Ruben and Gabriela have in feederism, and because of Grayson's significant involvement in two interviews. The next four interviews featuring Saskia, Gemma, Benny, and Gavin follow the interview schedule more closely and do not involve any professional interest. Their responses clustered around four themes: the meaning of feederism and early experiences; the meaning of food; secrecy; and extreme aspects of feederism.

Saskia

Meaning of feederism and early experiences

Saskia describes feederism in a fairly succinct way, saying that it is sexual attraction to fat people or people getting fatter. She describes herself as a mutual gainer with both feedee and feeder tendencies but has been exclusively a feedee in the past. Saskia feels that feederism can be done alone and that it is not necessary to have a feeder to gain weight and enjoy it. She describes being sexually interested in weight gain and says that "it's something that arouses me to an extent that is completely indescribable. I've actually found that I cannot be aroused by anything other than feederism stories or photos of people gaining weight." The strength of Saskia's attraction to weight gain is very clear.

In common with other participants, Saskia describes very early memories of fat fascination and describes being aged four and stuffing her clothes with pillows so that she would look fat. She also cites the expansion of Violet Beauregard in *Willy Wonka and the Chocolate Factory* as a fascinating image to her. At age 9 or 10, she describes waking up an hour and a half before everyone else in the house so that she could gather lots of food to take to her bedroom and eat it. She would then "have a double order breakfast as well, with the intent of gaining weight." Her first two romantic relationships at age 11 and 13 were with "quite chubby" partners whose excess weight attracted her. At school Saskia was bullied for gaining weight and claims that she never imagined her future partner as a thin person but as someone who was always much larger than her. Saskia's fascination with fat appears to be lifelong.

DOI: 10.1057/9781137470461.0006

The meaning of food

Saskia describes her current eating behaviour as being fairly continuous, snacking from 9 a.m. until 3 a.m. each day. She currently weighs about 270 lbs. and is working towards being 320 lbs. To do this, she tries to eat about 4,000 calories per day and is very aware of the calorie content of different foods. Saskia is indifferent to the taste of food and is happy to make 3500-calorie gainer shakes with no regard for how they taste. Sometimes Saskia is "able to eat for pleasure" but mostly she has calorie-related goals that take precedence. Attitudes towards the taste of food vary across our participants, but it is more common for participants to report enjoying food than to discuss it in such an instrumental way.

Secrets

Saskia has only told two or three people that she in is involved in feederism. She is very comfortable with her own body and enjoys it, but she also feels a pressure to fit in and conform, which she acknowledges is difficult as an almost 300-pound woman. She would be uncomfortable with everybody knowing about her participation in feederism. Being secretive about feederism for fear of being judged is common across the sample.

Extremes

Saskia's attitude to immobility and force-feeding is well-developed, and she has discussed the idea with feeders online. She is interested in being fed to immobility and also feeding another person to that level. For most participants, immobility is a fantasy-only concept, but Saskia is ready to go for immobility if the conditions are right. The main concern for her is a financial one and knowing that she would be cared for. The lack of freedom that would come with immobility is not mentioned. Helplessness is arousing to Saskia, and she describes how she would feel presiding over someone else reaching immobility: "rendering someone completely helpless, you know, to the point of which they can't even sit up by themselves in the morning, that's definitely a huge fantasy and something that I would strongly participate in." Saskia also finds the idea of tube-feeding and funnel-feeding "extremely erotic," and has taken part in force-feeding. She describes an incident in a previous relationship where she was tied up and forced to eat until the other person was satisfied.

DOI: 10.1057/9781137470461.0006

Gemma

Meaning of feederism and early experiences

Gemma defined feederism as people being attracted to the idea of gaining weight either for sexual purposes or because it feels better to be fatter. For most of her life she has identified as a feeder but her identity has gradually changed over the years and she now feels it would be more appropriate to be labelled as mutual gainer or a feedee. Gemma is currently in a relationship with a man who is not interested in feederism but would not mind if she started to gain weight (currently she is trying to lose weight). Gemma feels that she definitely does not need another person in order to be involved in feederism because gaining feels good in itself and she can feel attractive by herself.

As with most other participants, Gemma's interest in fat started at age three or four. She would fantasize about growing up to be "a really fat woman," and she thought the fat women she saw in public were very attractive. She first started to get sexual feelings towards fat women at around 11 or 12 years old and goes on to say that her attraction to fat is "pretty much a lifelong thing." Unprompted, Gemma suggested that feederism was "like a sexual orientation like homosexuality or heterosexuality ... but it's like a secondary orientation." This is a concept that will be discussed throughout this research. Gemma's first romantic relationship was at age 17 with a 260-pound woman who was one of the bigger girls in her school. Most of Gemma's relationships have been with large women, and she describes her former fiancé as a 360-pound woman. Gemma says that she "felt like a feeder" for long time and possessed a "double standard" where, despite her attraction to big women, she felt that she would become "unattractive, ugly, and unhappy" if she were to gain weight herself. The potential reasons for this emerge later in the interview, when Gemma discusses the fat phobia which she believes to be present within society generally, within the LGBT community, and within her own family. Gemma describes her mother as a vegan, body-conscious yoga teacher, and she feels this caused her problems in adjusting to herself as a feedee over the years.

The meaning of food

When Gemma is being a feedee, she eats large meals and snacks throughout the day. She describes herself as a "foodie" and says that she really enjoys good food and that the taste is important. She would not

DOI: 10.1057/9781137470461.0006

eat something just because of its high calorie value. This contrasts with a small number of participants who are very calorie-focused to the exclusion of all else. Gemma is a former vegetarian who still does not eat red meat. She says that she tries to be health-conscious and eat a healthy diet, but just eats a lot of food. Gemma acknowledges the difficulty of being a feedee and simultaneously remaining healthy, but she tries her best to do this.

Secrets

Gemma keeps feederism "very private." She has only told her best friend and boyfriend that she is involved in feederism, and her main reason for doing this is her perception of fat phobia. This is similar to other participants, who typically hide their interest from the majority of people.

Extremes

Gemma reports that she has not seen the documentaries made about feederism that depict some of the more extreme varieties of it (e.g. feeding to immobility). She has heard about them, though, and believes them to be "universally terrible." The depiction of women as victims in the documentaries bothers her as she believes they are designed for sensationalism and to have the shock value of "Jerry Springer." Gemma is very certain that female feedees *want* to be fed and that documentaries neglect the different gender and sexuality dynamics present in feederism.

Despite her dislike of extreme depictions, Gemma is very aware of force-feeding, and tube- and funnel-feeding. She thinks they sound exciting and fit with her interest in BDSM. Gemma likes to be tied up and forced to do things, but she does not feel she could trust someone to force-feed her as it would be "scary to put your wellbeing in someone else's hands." She also thinks that immobility "sounds incredibly exciting" and she would like to be on either the giving or receiving end of it. As with many participants, it is a potent fantasy for Gemma, but the reality of it has a challenging side that acts as a deterrent. Gemma thinks it would be awful in real life to have to see someone unable to function.

Benny

Benny provided written answers first and then took part in an interview. His analysis includes his answers from both sources.

DOI: 10.1057/9781137470461.0006

Meaning of feederism and early experiences

Benny identifies as a feeder, feedee, and mutual gainer. He has never had a specific feederism relationship, partly because he finds it hard as a heterosexual man to find a female feeder. Benny's experience of the feederism community is that most men who want to gain are gay. He describes his online profiles as generating a lot of comments and attention from gay men but very little from women. He says "the feederism community is full of fat, lonely straight guys who can't find women who either want to get fat or want to help them get fat". He believes that feederism is a male-dominated fetish and even suggested further research on feederism in the gay community.

Benny describes having a fascination with fat since childhood. He remembers at age 5 having a strong interest in a story about a pig that gained a large amount of weight, and he also mentions the cartoon *Pigs is Pigs* (discussed earlier). Throughout his childhood, he was very interested in stories about people who had gained weight or who were very heavy. Benny notes that he was a late developer sexually, saying that he didn't begin to masturbate until he was 20 and that the first time he kissed a girl was during his freshman year at college (approximately 18 years old). At school he would have crushes on slim girls but describes them as non-sexual crushes where he would just imagine holding hands or kissing the girl but never having sex. When he got to college he began to find bigger women sexy, especially if they gained weight. He illustrates this with an example of a girl he worked on a science project with who gained 30 lbs. over a summer. This made her very sexy and erotic to Benny, and he realized the transformation was a key arousing factor for him. One way in which transformation can be highlighted is by women wearing clothes that are too small for them because of their weight gain. Benny describes the sight of straining clothes as very arousing.

This links to a strong autoerotic element in Benny's feederism. He finds his own weight gain highly arousing, and he attributes this to the resulting feminization of his body. He describes his body as becoming more soft and developing breasts. When Benny bought his first bra to accommodate his growing breasts, he found it "a big turn on" and he describes wearing it with other women's clothes that are too small for him while he masturbates. His fantasies during masturbation typically involve moderate weight gain (e.g. 10 lbs.), but afterwards Benny resolves not to actually gain this amount of weight.

DOI: 10.1057/9781137470461.0006

Secrets

Benny reports only having told his brother that he specifically enjoys gaining weight but he has told more people that he likes bigger women. He doesn't think that his fetish is particularly bad, and he has found people to be open-minded about it when he has discussed liking big women. He describes the reaction of a woman he studied with as reassuring when she said, "Oh my God, that's hardly even a fetish anymore!" Benny sometimes doubts the integrity of people's face-to-face comments because of the very unpleasant comments he reads online underneath YouTube videos posted by gainers. He believes that people are more polite face-to-face and find it easier to say what they really think anonymously online.

Extremes

Benny has never wanted to be immobile even in his "wildest fantasies." This is quite different to many participants, who are happy to entertain the idea of immobility as a fantasy if they had unlimited wealth. Benny's opinion of immobility is that it is "incredibly bizarre that people would give up all the things life has to offer purely for sexual gratification." He also doesn't fantasize about being excessively large. Benny volunteers his dimensions as 6'3" and 270 lbs. (a BMI of 33) but he has no desire to get into the 300-pound+ range, which he feels is a common fantasy that is discussed a lot online. Benny also rejects the idea of tube-, funnel-, and force-feeding and wishes to distance himself from the BDSM aspect of feederism. He wants women to "feel sexy and beautiful" about their size and he is not happy addressing the masochistic interests of female feedees. He describes a situation online where a female feedee wanted him to pretend to be her doctor and tell her she was a "fat pig" who he couldn't treat until she lost weight. Benny is not comfortable with these scenarios.

Benny also finds mainstream depictions of feederism troubling. He feels that the main focus is on the idea of a man seeking out a woman to fatten up and make immobile. Typically the woman is somehow tricked or convinced to do this against her will. Benny described the film *Feed* (2005, discussed in Chapter 1) which tells the story of a police officer trying to track down a man who is feeding women to death. He finds this narrative of the man as an abuser inaccurate and unfair and distances himself from this portrayal.

DOI: 10.1057/9781137470461.0006

Gavin

Gavin is currently studying to be a nurse, and he also teaches anatomy and physiology. His stepfather was an orthopaedic surgeon, and Gavin has struggled to reconcile his arousal to weight gain with his medical knowledge of the effects of obesity. He is very aware of the Health at Every Size agenda but tries to keep a balanced view and not simply find ways to convince himself that his interests are healthy.

Meaning of feederism and early experiences

Gavin describes feederism as being when a person is attracted to their partner gaining weight and they help their partner do this by feeding him or her. He sees feederism mostly from the feeder perspective and identifies as a feeder. Despite this, Gavin does not believe it is necessary to have a feedee partner in order to participate in feederism. He has gone for long periods of time without a partner and is happy to masturbate to fantasies and images of feedees gaining.

Gavin's earliest memory of being interested in bigger women is somewhat later than many other participants. Gavin was 12 years old and started to use his computer to make animated drawings of women who would expand until their clothes came off. He was very secretive about this and says he would have been "mortified" if these animations had been discovered. When he was growing up, his mother was constantly on a diet and attended the gym five or six times a week. One of the ways in which he says feederism is thrilling is that it involves a woman "enjoying herself... she's lazy, hedonistic, enjoys pleasure. I had a morbid fear of all of that when I was growing up." Gavin describes becoming very embarrassed at age 14 when he first experienced flirting and playing footsie with a large girl in a swimming pool. He felt his interest in big women was "bizarre" for a long time. He understood there to be something bad about fatness but he found it irresistible. He describes it as "thrilling, shocking, kind of obscene." Despite being very comfortable in describing his interest in feedees, Gavin has wished he did not have such an interest many times. He believes that some women are repulsed by his interest in gaining. After a long-distance relationship with a 380-pound internet model from Canada who was happy to gain and entertain fantasies, Gavin is now in a relationship with a woman who allows him to feed her but does not want to gain.

DOI: 10.1057/9781137470461.0006

Secrets

Since age 19 or 20, Gavin has increasingly "come out" a lot to friends and family including his mother. He started to do this in conversations where women were being criticized about weight gain. He would speak up for them declaring them to be "hot" as a way of gradually making it known that he preferred large women. He took a 220-pound woman home to meet his mother, which he said resulted in her being "mystified... surprised... miffed" at his choices but also unable to have rational objections. Gavin says he has not encountered any real hostility from the people he has told about his preferences.

Extremes

When asked about force-, tube-, and funnel-feeding, Gavin describes it as "an old tradition." He is very aware of material on it that is available online including special equipment (in part because of his medical background). He has enjoyed fantasizing about it in the past but feels it places the feeder in a very dominant role, which he is not comfortable with. He prefers to "nudge" women towards gaining by doing activities that involve food. Gavin finds the idea of immobility repellent and describes the physiological implications such as bed sores. He used to read immobility fantasy material when he was 17 but is now very much against it and makes a range of sounds indicating his disgust at the concept. He feels that documentaries on feederism are "aberrant" and their decision to show immobility and other extreme behaviours makes life hard for feeders and feedees, and causes people to think feederism is abusive.

Gavin describes two of his own fantasies to reiterate his dislike of forcing and immobility. His "spoiled princess fantasy" involves meeting the needs of a woman with a hedonistic and lavish lifestyle who dominates him by demanding he serves her food requirements. He describes this as a "heady co-dependence." He also fantasizes about the "scandalous and erotic" nature of a woman who gains weight through "the vicissitudes of life" until she is incredibly fat. Gavin's excitement seems to come from the idea of women giving in and letting themselves go, which appears to be the antithesis of his mother.

Ashley, James, and Blossom

The final three interviewees gave answers that provided more varied themes. These are explored individually with each participant.

DOI: 10.1057/9781137470461.0006

Ashley

Ashley was approached through Twitter to take part in the research, and she agreed. She has a Clips4Sale page selling feederism videos.

Role fluidity and limitations of the health frame

Ashley thought of her feederism choices as being dependent on her mood. It was not simply a matter of identifying as a feeder or a feedee, because both terms were appropriate at different times. The roles that were shared with a partner had to be different but it was entirely possible for Ashley to have a dominant feeder role in a sexual dynamic: "I don't usually think of myself as a feeder and a feedee. I don't think of myself as mutual gaining because I don't normally like both people gaining at once. It's kind of one or the other and I just kind of switch depending on my mood."

There is a clear sense of fluidity of sexual role play, and this participant seems to be able to cross the divide quite easily. These roles have been depicted previously as fixed, particularly in regard to women taking on more dominant roles and men taking on submissive positions. Interesting Ashley describes how she was once "strictly a feedee," but this changed over time. "Probably a lot of it had to do with how I gained weight, and then I got to a point where it wasn't going to be fun to gain more, like it was too much work. And then I found out I had a slightly high blood sugar and I decided I wanted to fix that, and then just kind of switched over to enjoying other people gaining and not just my own. I just tried to balance it." This shows the degree of agency within feederism and also the level of education about food choices and health risks. Ashley also remarks that she does not stuff herself with food because "I know I inherited my mother's genes for diabetes so I just don't do it as much." This shows that the heath frame is not sufficient to deter people from engaging in feederism. Ashley does not lack knowledge about food and health; she assimilates the information and adapts her role in feederism accordingly. This suggests that the pull of feederism is strong and that it is hard for people to just stop taking part in it.

Commercial autoeroticism

Ashley understood her role fluidity as being selfish, in that she was mostly concerned with fulfilling her own desires at that particular time, but at the same time said that she had gained weight by herself in private. Gaining weight deliberately at home where nobody else is watching is consistent with many of our participants who describe autoerotic feeding. There was also

DOI: 10.1057/9781137470461.0006

a commercial aspect to this individualized weight gain as Ashley explains: "Now when I do it, I actually have a Clips4Sale site that I sometimes make a little money on, not much but that's mostly why I have a Tumblr now". Websites are used as a way of socializing and networking but when it comes to the exchange of money, Ashley describes the exchange as being one-sided, in that the interactions are dull and tedious, so she typically does not engage anymore, other than posting videos. "I actually make it so they just buy the clips and I never really actively interact with them." Engagement in feederism communities has become less about social engagement and more about posting content online for anonymous users to buy and exchange. The excitement and novelty of interaction is no longer a factor for Ashley.

Early experiences and family life

Like other participants, Ashley has been intrigued by fatness from an early age. "I've always had the inclination as young as I can imagine basically. I can remember watching Charlotte's Web and the Timpleton goes to the Fair and when he stuffs his face and gets fat, I was like wow this is the greatest sequence ever in movies, when I was like 7".

Ashley has not told her family about her involvement in feederism but suspects that her mother knows: "My mum probably knows, like she saw my Fantasy Feeder account once when she got on my computer and she pretends like she has no idea that she knows, even though one time she said something about it." She describes a pivotal moment in her childhood where she found a pile of her father's pornography magazines and that they were about larger women. "There was one that obviously had naked women with food on them and like what their favourite foods were and how much they weigh." She goes on to say, "I remember seeing them when I was like 13. I literally saw them in a stack and I saw that they weren't thin women and I opened one page and then I ran away and never saw them again. And then I saw them again like three years ago and that's when I actually looked in and saw the detailed images that actually are really similar to what I really like." Ashley was initially scared of this pornography and never explored it more in depth because she recognized that her sexual feelings "were not mainstream" even at 13 years old.

Food as a means to an end

Ashley's attitude towards food itself is not unique, but it is different to the majority of participants. The taste and smell of food does not matter to her: "Food is either fuel or something that makes people fat. I mean, honestly,

DOI: 10.1057/9781137470461.0006

I don't really care about food that much. For sexual reasons, it's necessary." Food is significant sexually, as a means to an end. This attitude is expected in those who favour tube- and funnel-feeding but is more unusual in those who eat conventionally.

James

James finds the weight gain of others attractive, so one would expect him to identify as a feeder. This is not the case as James has had negative experiences with other feeders, and so he does not like referring to himself as a feeder. In common with some other participants, he does not like the connotations that the term has and dislikes the association with abuse and psychological torment. James's responses are themed and he requested his name not be altered.

Early experiences

James's first awareness of his interest in weight gain at age 17 is later than most other participants. The interest developed with his first girlfriend (who was not interested in feederism) and James does not describe the childhood interest in fat that most other participants highlight. James describes his first awareness and experience of his sexual interest in feederism as scary: "So I suppose that would be my first experience with it, the first time that I found out that it was a part of me and it was really really scary." It was something "inside him" that made his relationship uncomfortable, like he was betraying his loved one. "I never attempted to control her and force her to gain weight, but at the same time, I still have that desire. I still wanted to see her gain weight. And it tore me apart. Here I am on the one hand, I love this woman with all my heart, I would give anything for her and on the other hand I don't even have enough control over myself. It was extremely frustrating." James found it difficult to express what it is about weight gain or bigger women that he finds attractive "asking a question like that is much like asking the question 'why do you like the colour yellow' or 'why do you enjoy going on drives at night-time.'" He described it as one of the "inherent properties of the human soul." The intensity of James's association with feederism is quite potent despite his late age in realizing it.

Family conflict and hedonism

When James asked to take part in this research he was initially going to be interviewed alongside his current feedee partner, but days before the interview

DOI: 10.1057/9781137470461.0006

happened, his partner decided not to participate, and there were difficulties in the relationship. This conflict arose due to James telling his parents about his interest in feederism. James remarked, "The way that they thought of it, they thought of me as a person who was going to enable her [his partner] in an unhealthy lifestyle and to ultimately have malicious intent for her." The problem was that the conventional frame of feederism as enabling a coercive relationship dynamic was troubling for his parents to accept. James relayed the conflict he had with his parents to his partner, who decided that she could not be with someone whose parents thought like that. The need for James to feel as though his sexual preferences were verified and accepted by his parents suggests a coming out, unveiling a hidden sexuality. James notes, "They flat out told me, if you had not brought this up to us, we would have never known." People are unaware of feederism's existence, according to James, and so they immediately react with hostility when hearing of it for the first time because of the counterintuitive ways in which sexuality and food are entwined.

When it came to secrecy, James said that he was tired of keeping it to himself. "I don't want to be hiding anymore. I've done the hiding, I've tried cutting it out, I've tried attempting to not be a feedist and it doesn't work." Feederism is not chosen, but he feels he can link it to his own personal philosophy. "I view being casual and taking things as they come and living in a hedonistic fashion where you simply enjoy yourself and enjoy the moment, enjoy what you're going to do be doing, what you're really doing and be at peace with yourself as opposed to trying to make yourself better." In this section, James talks about hedonism and about lifestyle choices that are focused on living in the moment, and his feederism links into this particular strand of Dionysian thought, where sensations and emotions regardless of the social revulsion they provoke should be in the open if they make people happy. He believes that there are merits to feederism, and he wants to show the general public what these merits are.

Blossom

Placing oneself

Blossom noted that every time she starts a conversation with someone she has met online, there is always a conversation about what terms are appropriate and how you would define yourself as someone in the community. Blossom (in common with some other participants) likes the term 'feedism' and the reason for this was the neutrality it conveyed. For her, feederism has connotations that suggest a one-sided relationship where power was vested

DOI: 10.1057/9781137470461.0006

in one partner over another. There is a benefit to being neutral, and opportunities for networking and creating contacts socially through feederism websites becomes easier. Blossom says she is "on the fence" when it comes to the terminology within feederism, and she classes her weight gain as an independent act, but also as a gainer. There is a clear sense that identifying yourself through terminology has intense thought associated with it. It is important enough to be the starting point of every online exchange Blossom has had. Blossom believed that feederism could be something done as an autoerotic act, and everything she has ever done has been "completely" on her own and for her own reasons.

Early experiences

Blossom recalls one of her earliest memories when she was 7 years old: "I was stuffing my shirt full of like plush stuffed animals and pretending I was outrageously fat. I remember it because one of my siblings walked in on me and caught me and it was mortifying."

She also recalls being fascinated with her mother's friend who was pregnant at an early age and finding the growing stomach particularly interesting. "I remember feeling a little embarrassed because I was so fascinated by the way that her belly expanded through her pregnancy." Blossom was particularly reflexive about this and remarked that it had nothing to do with the pregnancy itself, but rather the shape of her stomach. Blossom did not make this revelation though until later as she thought that instead of having an interest in weight gain, that it was an interest in pregnancy. She did not realize that it was a desire for weight gain until she found information about it on the internet; she was not previously exposed to the appropriate frame.

Dark side of the internet exchange and authenticity

Blossom discussed the problems with fake profiles on websites like fantasyfeeder.com. She notes, "What they do is, people will create a profile, they'll either put minimal information or pictures that look like they're from, you know google, they'll ask you to webcam chat, but they'll say that their's doesn't work and that they have no audio. That is somebody trying to pretend they're somebody else so they can have whatever sort of encounter with you. But then there are cases where people have gone onto that website and then post it on other sites. There's Reddit hate forums and tumblr is full of nasty re-postings of people saying awful things [...] It's a big risk to put yourself out there. I think as someone who's had that betrayed, it's very easy to feel quite cynical." Blossom feels very vulnerable about herself on the

DOI: 10.1057/9781137470461.0006

internet because of the negativity that exists outside the feederism community. The fetish is marginalized and treated in a negative way by others, and sometimes people are tricked into role-playing, only to have themselves recorded and placed on a different website. There is a sense that authenticity is a major anxiety in the feederism community both for accurate portrayals of feeders and feedees, and the diversity that exists, but also unease within the community about fake profiles and being taken advantage of by others.

Blossom discusses the scepticism that first arose when the current study came to her attention. "You know it does take a bit of trust, a lot of people were quite sceptical of your study. I posted about it on that website and yeah, I think the work of other researchers has actually left quite a bad taste in people's mouths."

Couples

Three couples were interviewed for the current research. Virginia and Terrance were interviewed in real time using Skype and gave a very long interview in excess of two hours. Dorothy and Dwight were interviewed in the same way but gave a shorter interview that was more similar to the third couple, Wendy and Reginald. Wendy and Reginald were the only participants to be interviewed face-to-face, and they visited Edinburgh Napier University to take part in the research. The interviews were analysed using thematic analysis.

Virginia and Terrance

Virginia and Terrance gave a long interview in excess of two hours, and their responses revealed different themes to the other two couples so their data are analysed separately. Their responses centred on authenticity and health narratives.

Definitions and authenticity

Virginia defined feederism in a relational way, whereby growing larger was assisted by the presence of a partner. She recognized that this was a narrow definition but felt this was the bones of the definition. She goes on to say that she views herself as having a broad range of different fat- and weight-related kinky behaviours. There is a sense that feederism is defined by the person, the identifier is entirely subjective to encompass a range of different behaviours which might come be part of the master theme. This sense of locating oneself and having a sense of authenticity became a significant focus of the

DOI: 10.1057/9781137470461.0006

interview, particularly when looking at feederism as a distinct and novel sexuality when compared to other forms of fat admiration and fetishism. Terrance notes, for example, "Just liking someone with large bellies does not make you a feeder or liking someone who's eaten so much their stomach is rumbling, that is very much a separate interest." The difference is that feederism is always distinct because it "focuses on either literally manifesting the weight gain or creating imaginary situations or role play situations that still focus on the actual growth in gaining."

Healthy narratives: childhood and beyond

Virginia remembers her first experience of wandering through an unfamiliar city with her parents at six years old and seeing a sign in a pharmacy window that was advertising a weight-loss product. She remembers being transfixed by the sign due to the way it depicted fat, and she remembers distinctly hanging back from her family in order to look at the sign more. The intended narrative of the sign was to encourage and reinforce healthy living and dieting, which was a common experience that Virginia had growing up. Food was particularized in her household with a considerable emphasis on healthy living and eating. Her mother cooked all of their meals and took care to ensure that the food was nutritious and balanced. This highly controlled experience of growing up led to what Virginia called "unstructured snacking" when she went to university. It was liberating to be able to eat whenever she wanted, and she started to experiment with food and sexuality. Calorie counts are placed on restaurant menus with the idea of informing people about healthy eating choices, but this has become an easy way for Virginia to deliberately choose meals that contain the highest levels of fat. She remarks, "I find it extremely arousing and, you know, I know that it's intended to cause people to think twice whether they really need a main dish that has 2,000 calories in it. But I on the other hand find myself looking at the menu and going, 'oh good, this one has got 2,000 calories, that's great.'" Healthy eating messages have had the opposite effect, and instead of encouraging a compliance with the dominant narratives which encourage fit and skinny bodies, it was a way of seeing an opposite which appealed to Virginia in her childhood and a way of maintaining her gaining now. It was seeing her desires in a pathologized representation of the body. This sense of deviancy was experienced on the individual level; it was performed. Virginia felt her way around this body by padding. She used to pad her pyjamas with pillows as a child, which continued into her teenage life. It was done for erotic reasons but also acted as a fantasy because Virginia could see herself fatter.

DOI: 10.1057/9781137470461.0006

This symbiosis of fantasy and reality was realized through popular culture such as cartoons, novels and advertising but also through her own elaborate performances of fat. Fat was rehearsed and played with in private, which allowed a feeling-out process that combined with a sense of sensuality in feeling the padding on her own stomach.

Fat was well-known to be deviant by Virginia and was seen and experienced as a deviation from a standard societal norm of slender and fit bodies from her early life. This was mainly due to the ways in which fat bodies were invisible. When other girls were transfixed by celebrity culture and were pinning posters on their walls, Virginia remembers being enthralled by fat. Virginia grew up pre-internet and so was unable to find solace and comfort in the experiences of like-minded people on forums until she was in her 20s. These experiences therefore constitute a piecing together of one's identity through disparate sources, often in serendipitous ways. When she was a teenager, she remembers finding a book in a library sale, where they were getting rid of books they no longer needed. It was a novel that included scenes of a young boy who was enslaved and "fattened up" and she remembers this as the most erotic things she had ever read.

When she was younger, it was very difficult for her to admit that she had a sexual attraction to larger people and was afraid of rejection with thin people being seen as "morally superior," more successful and more attractive generally. Terrance discussed the fascination he had as a child with transformations on a sexual and non-sexual level. The transformation of the body external to him was fascinating, and he remembers cartoons that involved women getting bigger, which is a recurring theme in our sample as a whole with popular culture being a stimulus.

"Pigs is Pigs" as a Cultural artefact

When asked about the cartoon "Pigs is Pigs," Terrance remarked that it was impossible to be active in the weight gaining community in the late 1990s or early 2000s without dozens of people mentioning the cartoon. The cartoon was mentioned in retrospective fashion with many watching it later in life. Virginia explains, "It was not formative to me but to the authors of many of the weight gain erotic stories that I first encountered, it was very formative." He described watching it as being like seeing an artefact that affected a culture that he was a part of. It was like going to an art museum and seeing a piece of work that you are not moved by particularly but you recognize that the artist in question has influenced some of your favourite painters. This description shows that certain pieces of popular culture are canonized

DOI: 10.1057/9781137470461.0006

within the subculture, in being a staple for showcasing a certain archetype that is consistent throughout a lot of the fantasy fiction in the community, that of the growing and expanding body.

Reginald and Wendy; Dorothy and Dwight

These two couples gave interviews of a similar length, and key themes for both were the understanding of feederism as a fetish or sexuality, and agency in feederism.

Fetish/sexuality

Traditionally sexuality is understood in terms of sexual orientation relating to a person's gender (e.g. heterosexual, homosexual, bisexual). More recent terminology has evolved that reflects more diverse understandings of sexuality and gender identity (e.g. pansexual to describe a person who is essentially gender-blind and may be attracted to either gender or to a person who identifies as neither male nor female (Jones & Hill, 2008)). Nevertheless, the term "sexual orientation" is still focused on ideas of gender and is assumed as a baseline on which other sexual interests or preferences are built. A sexual *preference* suggests choice, whereas sexual orientation is considered by many to be biologically determined (Frankowski, 2004) and fairly stable. Sexualities that do not conform to these gender-based understandings tend to be regarded as paraphilia (e.g. bestiality). In contrast, a fetish can relate to anything and need not have any gender content (e.g. a rubber fetish). It may be sexual arousal based on textures, individual body parts, inanimate objects, or on restraints for example. A fetish can be seen as an addition to a person's sexuality.

Although there are technical definitions of fetishes and sexuality which vary slightly across academic disciplines, there is also a broad understanding of these terms which can be inferred from the interviewees. Essentially a fetish is seen by participants as something that is chosen, that is dynamic, and that may develop at any time. Conversely a sexuality is seen as something that has always been present, is fixed, is not chosen, and is an integral part of a person's character or identity. Although these definitions do not map onto official definitions they are still useful in understanding how participants experience feederism. Participants often borrowed from the language of homosexuality by describing themselves "coming out" as a feeder/feedee, being afraid to "come out," as having a "deviant sexuality," and speculating on whether there was therapy for feederism for people who did not want to live with it just as there is the

DOI: 10.1057/9781137470461.0006

highly controversial conversion therapy purporting to "cure" homosexuality. When participants were asked to discuss what feederism meant to them, they spontaneously began to describe it as a fetish:

> "it's just a fetish involving overeating" (Reginald)
>
> "some sort of fetish or erotic feeling towards fat" (Wendy)
>
> "I definitely think it's a fetish" (Dorothy)
>
> "anything involving any aspect of the fetish, anything from weight gain to the feeding process" (Dwight)

Over the course of the interviews, the participants changed their minds and began to describe feederism as a sexuality after initially rejecting this term and preferring fetish:

> "I can definitely relate to it being a sexuality, I consider it to be a sexuality, definitely" (Wendy)
>
> "in the broader fetish communities it never quite sits right" (Reginald)
>
> "it's like many other facets of human sexuality" (Dwight)

This shift over the course of the interview may have occurred as a result of describing early life experiences where a pre-pubertal interest in fat and weight gain was evident. Describing these feelings and experiences may have cemented the idea in participants' minds that they had not chosen feederism and therefore it had more in common with a stable sexuality than a dynamic fetish.

> "I was really really really young. Like three or four and my neighbour that lived next door ... was a super fat lady and I thought she was so pretty and I wanted to be like her" (Dorothy)
>
> "when I was really young I realised, oh I want to be really fat because I thought it was super sexy. Probably like around 10 or 11" (Dorothy)
>
> "they had one where Babs Bunny is, some enemy of hers hypnotizes her and forces her to eat carrot cake until she like can't move, and I just remember being like five and being like I feel funny" (Dwight)
>
> "when I was pretty young, probably about 12, I remember I did come across like stories and stuff online, so like it's always been an interest" (Wendy)

Participants also clearly linked their feederism to their sense of self or identity as can be seen in Wendy and Dwight's words.

> "It's part of my identity" (Wendy) "it's part of who I am, it's always sort of going to be there" (Wendy) "I didn't really feel like I had a sexuality until ... I discovered that this is what I was into" (Wendy)
>
> "it's not really a choice that people make" (Dwight)

DOI: 10.1057/9781137470461.0006

Agency

Another important theme that emerged early in the interviews was agency. Asking participants what terminology they preferred to describe themselves (e.g. feeder, feedist, feedee) often elicited wider comments on what different terms meant to different people. Issues of consent and desire were key in determining the terms individuals preferred. Wendy was very keen to demonstrate her agency at several points in the interview and it was clearly important to her to show that she didn't just consent to being a feedee; she actively enjoyed the role and sought out opportunities to embrace it. She also wanted to distinguish feedee from gainer, as she was not deliberately trying to gain weight –, rather she was indifferent to the inevitable weight gain that would result from her behaviour:

> "I don't like force feeding. I like it to come from me, I like it to be my own gluttony. Yeah it's all about me" (Wendy)
>
> "It's your self-indulgence that's really attractive" (Reginald)
>
> "I think it's all me" (Wendy) "I would much rather talk about how fat I actually am" (Wendy)

Dorothy also identified as a feedee yet portrays this in a very different way. The desire is still evident but she adopts a much more submissive attitude:

> "it's just really hot to me. It's an act of submission. I think it's the greatest act of submission ... complete submission and I just find it super sexy" (Dorothy)
>
> "I like food. I like everything about it. So food, in and of itself, is like super erotic and the outcome is awesome" (Dorothy)

Both women describe being a feedee differently, yet both clearly show agency. The idea that female feedees are tricked or forced into their role does not come across in these accounts of being a feedee. In both cases the role appears to be enjoyed and embraced. The other side of this dynamic is that Reginald takes a more submissive role as a 'feedist' (a term he prefers over 'feeder'):

> "It's very sensual, it's very sort of luxurious and that's very erotic" (Reginald)

Dwight on the other hand performs a more dominant role in his relationship with Dorothy:

> "We've done tube feeding and ... light force feeding" (Dwight).
>
> "immobility is the goal. It's something that will take years and require a great deal of planning, but it's something we're definitely doing in real life" (Dwight)

DOI: 10.1057/9781137470461.0006

Section 1

Part 3 – Summary of themes

Although there were differences between interviewees, with some having had much more involvement and experience of feederism, there were also some similarities in the way participants answered the questions. After analysing the 23 participants in this study, three super themes have been identified: early attraction to fat; agency; and fantasy. Other themes emerge in different interviews, but these three themes are common across the data. The interview questions focused on some of these topics, so it was inevitable they would emerge – what is more interesting is the similarity of answers across participants.

Childhood interest in fat begins as early as four years old in some participants, with others unable to recall the age at which it began. For some, the interest is visual (e.g., watching films and cartoons, looking at pictures, or looking at people), and for others the interest becomes a performance where they stuff toys and pillows into their clothes and fantasize about expansion. Some participants describe overweight relatives feeling good to hug. In a small number of participants, the interest in fat began in later childhood (age 11 onwards), which is likely to coincide more with puberty. These participants talk more of secret eating and attraction to other children who were overweight. All participants became aware of their interest in fat before the age of 18.

The issue of agency was important in this research because previous portrayals of feederism focused on domination and lack of control for the feedee. Mainstream depictions particularly encouraged this belief, whilst academic analysis also centred on patriarchy and psychopathology. The interviewees in this research presented a very different picture with agency at the heart of how they talked about themselves and feederism. Every single participant emphasized choice, and this was done in a variety of ways. In addition to describing practical issues around choice in sexual behaviours, many participants also talked in detail about the language of feederism and the assumptions around particular words. Although this research has used the terms feederism, feedee, and feeder, most participants rejected these and preferred subtle variations that eliminated the implied power dynamic (e.g. feedist rather than feeder, feedism rather than feederism). Several participants also expressed their concern about non-consensual depictions of feederism and wanted to

DOI: 10.1057/9781137470461.0006

emphasize their rejection of such behaviours. This was observed in both male and female participants, further challenging the idea that men wish to force women into becoming feedees.

A further way in which agency was explored was by participants raising the issue of which role was dominant in feederism. It has always been assumed to be the feeder, but this was also challenged by some participants who described situations and experiences of dominant feedees. This is also reflected in feederism: fantasies where feedees can make extraordinary demands on their feeder.

It is prudent to acknowledge that finding many examples of positive, consensual feederism does not negate the existence of a darker, coercive element. There is a strong element of humiliation in some feederism encounters. Grayson speaks of the combination of pleasure and humiliation that his interests cause him, and there is clearly a crossover into the blackmail/humiliation genre of sexual activity. The site Clips4Sale describes itself as an amateur porn and fetish porn site. It features a number of users who will produce video clips on request or who have an existing library that can be purchased by other users. Grayson describes a series of online encounters with a woman from this site who he claims eventually ended up blackmailing him into further weight gain. The site contains over 17,800 clips tagged with "feederism." One example is a 15-minute video available for $15.99 which purports to show a slim, submissive gay man being force-fed 10 cheeseburgers and then tied to a chair and fed a "gainer shake" through a funnel by his dominant partner. This harsher depiction of feederism certainly has a fan base along with other more potentially problematic aspects (e.g. a cross over into financial domination, where feedees demand money from an online feeder so that they can eat more food and gain more weight). Extreme pornography exists for all sexual interests, though, and this is where the link to the final theme of fantasy is interesting.

The issue of force-feeding, tube- and funnel-feeding, and immobility was discussed with all participants. Everyone interviewed was aware of these things through reading about them, watching videos, and in a small number of cases experimenting with them. For all participants (except Dwight) immobility was a fantasy. It was something to be imagined and toyed with but was considered dangerous and unrealistic in reality. Those who had experimented with force-feeding and tube-feeding had done so with staged forcing, so that the person receiving the food could end the procedure at any time. Although forcing and immobility appear in feederism fantasy and are fantasized about by participants, their real-life

DOI: 10.1057/9781137470461.0006

presence in this sample was virtually non-existent. As with the issue of agency, it is important to raise this, as immobility has often been used as a shocking promotional tool to generate prurient interest and revulsion towards feederism. Those involved in feederism generally have no interest in becoming immobile.

Section 2

Weight stories

The final analytical section of this chapter explores feederism fantasy related to weight gain. Fiction is very popular on a number of websites and this section explores five weight gain stories. Lewis (2011) notes that storytelling might be the principal way of understanding the lived world since stories are "both art and quotidian, centripetal and centrifugal, running deep and wide through the human psyche" (Lewis 2011, p.505). Storytelling helps us understand our own identities and the identities of others, which Lewis (2011) states are a type of symbiosis. We use the narratives in stories to help us establish our own personal life stories; we take props, ideas or characterization and apply them. Narrative has been used as a viable way of giving marginalized voices a space for expressing a more nuanced and complete social reality of their existence, and the feederism community uses stories as a way of communicating fantasies that are considered deviant in a safe online environment. Stories therefore act as a form of resistance and as a way of documenting what is unseen; de Certeau (1984), for example, suggests that stories can be a viable way of standing up against "instituted power."

Jung, in his conceptualization of the archetype, recognized the ways in which narrative helps structure ideas within fables, myths, parables and folktales. These archetypes run through the fictional content called "weight stories" that are posted online by members of the Feederism community. These stories typically involve extraordinary weight gain that is facilitated and enabled through other means.

Men gaining: female feeding stories

There is a sizable number of stories which focus on a man having a gaining role, usually submissive and subordinate to a more dominant female feeder.

DOI: 10.1057/9781137470461.0006

These stories sometimes have significant metaphysical elements and will often feature fantastical situations or characters.

In "Men Gaining," a story on the popular website *Dimensions*, a fantasy object is established in the first sentence, an elusive rumour is told in the third person about a man who is described as the "fattest man ever to have lived." The man lives next door, but along with the rumours of his massive size come a series of rumours about the inaccessibility and guarded nature of the man. It is speculated that he has vicious guard dogs and crazed family members who are armed with shotguns. The house is fortress-like and is surrounded by barbed wire fences with considerable acres of land from the wall up to the house. Fat here is seen as a desirable attribute that requires around-the-clock protection, to prevent voyeurism and unwanted attention from a gaze. The protagonists (Joe and Pete) of the story are also described as fat teenagers, but they are curious to see a larger man. They eventually look through the man's window after discovering that there was no intense security around the property and saw a "strange-off white and pinkish rounded thing." It is described as being as wide as a doormat and was spilling from one room to another. The strange object turns out to be part of the man and the focus therefore is abstracted. The body is not recognized at all as the focus is entirely on the spilling mass of fat. Fat therefore becomes a partialism, in that the fixation is purely based on the enormity of flesh. The flesh has no discernible attributes that isolate it as a particular part of the body; it is simply a mass. The flesh is also naked and thus exposed to the gaze of the protagonists. The boys enter the house (which is unlocked) and approach the man, who was apparently sleeping. His weight is fantasized and exaggerated massively and is described as being wall to wall, filling entire rooms. The man wakes up and immediately says to the boys, "I suppose I should tell you how I got like this since your curiosity was obviously enough to overwhelm your sense of manners." He asks the boys to climb on top of him and to make themselves comfortable. This type of hospitality is a type of forniphilia, which is making a person into a type of furniture. Fat in this story encompasses the entire home and so the body is now makeshift chairs.

The man begins to tell a fat story describing how he became large. He describes taking part in an archaeological dig unearthing an old pirate settlement in Florida that is 450 years old and finding a genie bottle. The genie is a vanishing mediator (Žižek, 2008) who helped the man gain weight by progressively allowing him to gain weight daily in small segments through literal wish fulfilment. The genie eventually becomes the man's lover and is

DOI: 10.1057/9781137470461.0006

present in the room but under the man's flesh, the genie effectively became a fantasy enabler in transforming the body and the fantasy element of the story is the externalized influence of the genie. The man watches himself grow larger and larger with next to no input. The story is unusual in the sense that it involves a man who has grown to an enormous size with two boys listening to the story like apprentices, the genie, who is female, is his enabler and is thus similar to the role of a female feeder.

In another story titled, "His Feeder," a man talks about meeting a plump woman named "Linda." He was quite slender, but he describes having an attraction to slightly larger women. Linda wants to lose 20 pounds, but he says that her weight is fine. Progressively it turns out that Linda enjoys force-feeding her partners and feeding them considerable amounts of food and convinces the man to gain massive amounts of weight. Weight gain is meticulously recorded on a chart. Linda eventually loses significant amounts of weight because of her focus on feeding the man. Her desire to eat is lost and externalized onto another body. He must eat to fulfil her desires, but critically, she uses him as a vehicle for her own food-related wants.

A story titled "The Feeder Within" involves a man called Greg who after a car accident wakes up in a medical research institute and has become a 300-pound woman. The research institute had performed a memory transfer to allow him to live, moving his memories onto a computer and placing them into the body of another. This type of gender symbiosis is interesting but also reflective of the ways in which women and fat are seen to more commonly go together. Fat is often feminized and muscle is seen as a masculine trait. The fat male body therefore is a marginalized type of masculinity and so the transformation of himself into a female is due to his weight gain. His masculinity died in the car crash, in other words.

Co-constructed fat

In a story titled "Getting Fat with Friends," a contest is created amongst three friends to see how fat they can become. They order bottles of "Gainmore2000" which supposedly allowed their stomachs to take an infinite amount of food and converted all calories into 100% fat. The physiological change in the body then is determined regardless of the food consumed, all food is somehow converted into fat stores through the consumption of this magical milkshake. At the end of the story, all three friends are as fat as each other but decide to continue eating anyway, a type of fat infinite regress, where fat is an ongoing

DOI: 10.1057/9781137470461.0006

process that is shared and experienced as a group. The enabler in this story is external again to the gainers –, expansion is through magic.

Fattest in the world

A common theme in these stories is impossible weight gain and size, particularly with the intention of being the fattest person in the world. As mentioned in the "Men Gaining" story, the man was billed as being the fattest person in the world, due to the influence of his mystical genie feeder. This boundlessness of the body is explored in many different stories. In the story, "Joy finds her guy," for example, Tom, the focus of the story, serendipitously receives a note in his office from someone asking to meet in a nearby cafe. The note makes it clear that the writer knows about Tom's desires, which are about feeding and watching women gain. Tom arrives in the café to see a woman who is at least 400 pounds and is wearing a tight dress which accentuates all of her fat folds. He proceeds to order her massive quantities of food, which she happily consumes with pleasure. The story climaxes with the woman (Joy) telling Tom that she wants to be a "thousand pounds of pure bliss" after Tom professed his love for her. Other stories feature women who expand to the size of the entire universe. These impossible scenarios allow the writer and reader to engage in a world where anything is possible, and as a result these stories tend to allow for extreme weight gain without the consequences of immobility, or health problems that come with such intense gaining. In "Men Gaining," for example, the genie expands the size of the man's organs and bones in order to allow his body to accommodate the sheer mass of fat that is gained.

Section 3

Conclusions

This chapter has presented an analysis of 23 participants who self-identify as being involved in feederism, along with five weight gain stories from *Dimensions Magazine*. Super themes of early interest in fat, agency, and fantasy have been identified resulting in both mainstream depictions and some academic work being challenged. The final chapter explores the contribution this research makes, the limitations of it, and the practical implications it has. Directions for future research in this area are also discussed.

DOI: 10.1057/9781137470461.0006

References

Connell, R. (2006). *Masculinities*. Berkley, CA: University of California Press.

De Certeau, M. (1984). *The Practice of Everyday Life*. Berkley, CA: University of California Press.

ExtremeFeeding (2014). Helping a Friend. Retrieved April 1, 2015, from http://extremefeeding.com/index.php/en/stories/item/583-helping-a-friend.

ExtremeFeeding (2015). Rubens Feeders Extreme Feeding: Helping You Getting Fatter Since 1999. Retrieved April 1, 2015, from http://extremefeeding.com/index.php/en/videos-en/itemlist/user/43-rubens_feeder.

Feabie (2015). Retrieved June 10, 2015, from http://www.feabie.com/.

Frankowski, B. L. (2004). Sexual Orientation in Adolescents. *Pediatrics, 113*, 1827–1832.

GBWR (2015). *Guinness Book of World Records: Largest Natural Breasts*. Retrieved May 30, 2015, from http://www.guinnessworldrecords.com/world-records/largest-natural-breasts.

Grommr (2015). Retrieved February 9, 2015, from http://www.grommr.com/.

Jones, B. E. & Hill, M. J. (2008). *Mental Health Issues in Lesbian, Gay, Bisexual, and Transgender Communities*. Washington, DC: American Psychiatric Publishing Inc.

Lewis, P. J. (2011). Storytelling as Research/Research as Storytelling. *Qualitative Inquiry, 17*, 505–510.

Monaghan, L. F. (2005). Big Handsome Men, Bears, and Others: Virtual Constructions of "Fat Male Embodiment". *Body & Society* 11, 81–111.

Prohaska, A. (2014). Help Me Get Fat! Feederism as Communal Deviance on the Internet. *Deviant Behavior, 35*, 263–274.

Robinson, M. D., Wilkowski, B. M., & Meier, B. P. (2008). Approach, Avoidance, and Self-Regulatory Conflict: An Individual Differences Perspective. *Journal of Experimental Social Psychology, 44*, 65–79.

Žižek, S. (2008). *In Defense of Lost Causes*. London: Verso.

DOI: 10.1057/9781137470461.0006

3
Future Directions for Feederism

Abstract: *The final chapter of this text offers a theoretical contribution that challenges conventional views in the literature, particularly the pathology narrative in psychology and the patriarchal coercion view in sociology. Practical applications of the research are discussed, which include educating medical staff to increase awareness of feederism and a shift in focus from weight loss towards physical health. Research on Health at Every Size and the "obesity paradox" is used to underpin these recommendations. Limitations of the current research are discussed along with recommendations for future studies. These recommendations include quantitative research and greater participant diversity.*

Charles, Kathy and Michael Palkowski. *Feederism: Eating, Weight Gain, and Sexual Pleasure.* Basingstoke: Palgrave Macmillan, 2015. DOI: 10.1057/9781137470461.0007.

Theoretical contribution

There is still no clear answer about what might *cause* feederism. Feederism exists on a continuum and the roles individuals adopt within it are dynamic. A person does not necessarily spend their whole life as a feeder or feedee. Those who took part in this research certainly appear to have a lifelong connection to fat, though. The most consistent finding across participants was an interest in fat and expansion from a very young age. If feederism is to be classified as a fetish (which is what many of the participants choose to call it, even though it does not relate to inanimate objects), psychological literature on fetishism should offer some insight into its origins. The earliest work on sexual fetishism generally takes a dim view of it and seeks to medicalize and pathologize. Pettinger (1993) outlines Alfred Binet's analysis of fetishism from the 1880s. Binet believed that fetishism originated from a chance encounter or incident in childhood that happened to be paired with sexual arousal and a tainted or flawed character. Pettinger's example from Binet is of a five-year-old boy getting his first erection when he saw an elderly relative put on a nightcap. For the rest of his life he had a fetish for nightcaps and could not get aroused without seeing or imagining them on an old woman. The man is described as coming from a "tainted family" and as an adult suffered from depression, thus demonstrating his flawed character. Binet believed that everyone is subject to chance encounters with objects and arousal in childhood, but only those with a degenerate disposition develop a fetish.

Apart from the language used, in many ways, little has changed in the psychological understanding of fetishes and unusual sexual behaviour. More recent understandings still consider fetishes to stem from emotional childhood incidents that become linked to sexual arousal. At the most basic level, the concept is behaviourist – the reinforcing pairing of desire with an image or sensation. Treatments for taboo and illegal desires have incorporated a significant amount of behaviourist principles since the 1950s. Bancroft and Marks (1968) outline their attempts to treat a variety of sexual "deviants" with electric aversion. These patients comprised homosexuals, paedophiles, sadomasochists, transvestites, and transsexuals. Despite the very mixed results (some of which could have been anticipated, e.g. their sadomasochistic patients experiencing *increased* erections during treatment) basic ideas from this approach have carried through into more modern treatments. Even cognitive-behavioural

DOI: 10.1057/9781137470461.0007

treatments such as covert sensitization are based on the same principles (Beech, Craig, & Browne, 2009). Sexual desires and fetishes are seen as learned and can therefore be un-learned through the same mechanisms if necessary. The idea of a tainted family or degenerate disposition has also been maintained through the more scientific approach of searching for hereditary aspects of sex offending (Långström, Babchishin, Fazel, Lichtenstein, & Frisell, 2015). As discussed in Chapter 1, the desire to categorize, medicalize, and pathologize sexual behaviours is relatively new. Although there might be broad agreement in Western cultures that rape, paedophilia, sadism, and other paraphilia and fetishes that may harm people should be contained and treated in some way, there is no reason why there should be agreement about other kinds of atypical sexuality.

In almost all cases, feederism is consensual and not harmful. It is still viewed as an atypical sexual practice for which both participants and outsiders seek an explanation. The current sample did not provide evidence of conscious memories or experiences as overtly sexual as the nightcap example provided by Binet. They did cite instances of early childhood fascination with fatness and/or expansion. The examples were not unusual or unique, e.g. the "Pigs is Pigs" cartoon, the expansion of Violet Beauregard in the film *Willy Wonka & the Chocolate Factory* (1971), seeing images of overweight women in magazines, and seeing overweight girls at school or in their neighbourhood. None of these examples are strange or rare – they are things that many thousands of other children will have also seen. Binet's theory would suggest that those who went on to become involved in feederism must somehow have a tainted or degenerate character. Leaving aside the dated language, there was no consistency among participants when it came to describing other aspects of their lives, such as mental illness, difficult family relations, or abuse. Some participants had experienced these things, but there was no pattern among participants.

It is perhaps more useful to look outside the 19th and 20th century perspectives on sexuality and try to appreciate the bigger picture. Castelo-Branco, Huezo, and Lagarda (2008) discuss the nature of human sexuality in the 21st century and argue that there are new forms of sexuality that are linked closely to technology (e.g. non-contact sex through webcams). They also go on to highlight the separation between sex and reproduction that is well underway in Western societies. Much of the earliest psychological research on sexuality considered sexual acts that

DOI: 10.1057/9781137470461.0007

did not lead to reproduction as deviant (e.g. masturbation, oral sex, and homosexuality). It took much of the 20th century for these ideas to be dismantled. It is no coincidence that sexual interest in non-genital body parts and inanimate objects is still considered pathological, even though such interests may not be harmful. The attraction to fat and expansion in most cases is not going to lead to reproduction, so feederism is an atypical sexuality in that sense. The desire for psychology to explain feederism as though it were a mental illness or defect is perhaps misplaced, though. A presumption of pathology dictates the form and direction of research as potentially limiting our understanding. Acknowledging feederism as an alternative kind of sexuality may help research develop a different focus which allows movement towards understanding and exploring, rather than explaining and fixing.

Limitations

The findings presented in the previous chapter are subject to a number of limitations. During the design of the research, it was anticipated that recruiting participants would be difficult because feederism is portrayed as taboo and a niche interest in the mainstream media. Previous research on feederism had also often avoided using samples of actual feeders and feedees, preferring instead to use online postings made on feederism websites. Research that did recruit participants typically had very small sample sizes and highlighted the difficulty of obtaining trust from feeders and feedees. As such, the current research anticipated recruitment difficulties and set about making the process as non-invasive as possible with a target of four interviewees. Being non-invasive meant that participants were not asked to disclose their age, gender, sexual orientation, or educational background. Whilst this sensitivity was appreciated by participants, several voluntarily provided much of the information during conversation or in their initial approach. Because this disclosure was not consistent, it led to an incomplete picture of the participants who took part in the study. After a very slow start, recruitment burgeoned and more than 20 participants were interviewed, with many more being turned away as the deadline for completing the research approached. In retrospect, most participants would have probably been happy to formally share

DOI: 10.1057/9781137470461.0007

more demographic information about themselves, and this would have allowed a clearer picture of the sample to be presented. It would have also been possible to carry out a small-scale quantitative study if the keenness for participation had been anticipated. There is currently no quantitative research on feederism, and this is an area for future research which will be explored later.

An implication of not having a full picture of participants' demographics is that it is not possible to know to what extent the current sample represents the general population or even the feederism community itself. As with all research that relies on voluntary participation without any reward, only certain types of people tend to come forward. Volunteerism tends to result in participants with higher levels of education and intelligence, higher social class, more arousal-seeking tendencies, tendency to be more sociable, more likely to be female, and lower on authoritarianism when compared to the general population (Wilson & MacLean, 2011). Taking part in this research required participants to commit to an interview time slot, to complete a number of forms, and to discuss in some detail their sexual interests and practices. It is not unreasonable to assume that many people would have considered that onerous or intrusive, so it would have been useful to know more about the people who came forward. Recruitment was also done entirely online as was participation (with the exception of one couple who were interviewed face-to-face), which also excludes some members of the community. Despite these concerns regarding participant demographics, it is evident from participants who volunteered information that there is a diverse range of age, sexuality, and gender, as well as roles (i.e. feeders, feedees, and mutual gainers).

Another participant-related limitation, which can affect any research focused on sexual behaviour, is that individuals who are in abusive and controlling relationships may have been unable or unwilling to take part is this study. None of the participants recruited for this research said that they were in genuinely coercive situations. Some described circumstances of coercion that they had orchestrated for their own pleasure, but none described a situation that could be considered abusive. The conclusion drawn from this is that the reality of feederism does not meet the mainstream portrayal of coercion and domination, but this could be an artefact of the sample obtained. Researchers should continue to be mindful of the potential unheard voices in feederism.

DOI: 10.1057/9781137470461.0007

Practical applications and implications

Although not everyone involved in feederism is obese, it is undeniable that for many it is an inevitable conclusion of long-term overeating. Some feedees are able to maintain the same weight and indulge in overeating periodically, but this is not the norm. Visceral fat and physical expansion are key sexual elements in feederism, and most feedees or mutual gainers appear to exist in the overweight or obese weight category. Several of the participants in the current research put limits on their weight gain for health and mobility reasons, but based on self-disclosed weights and body descriptions these limits are not within the normal weight range defined using Body Mass Index (BMI, WHO, 2015). BMI is a widely used approach for classifying a person's weight as underweight, normal, overweight, or obese (with the obese category having several classes reflecting increasing size). It is a simple calculation based on dividing mass by the square of height. The use of the BMI system to classify healthy weight has been debated for many years on two fronts. First, the cut-off for the overweight and obese categories varies in different countries, meaning that a person might be considered overweight in Japan but of a normal weight in the UK. Secondly, the science of the BMI itself has been criticized. BMI is a measure of the density of a person and does not provide any information on the composition of their body. This means that individuals with high muscle density are sometimes classified as obese despite having very little body fat. Oliver (2006) offers a detailed analysis of the problems with using BMI to classify obesity.

Concerns about growing rates of obesity are well-publicized globally and have been for some time. The World Health Organization reports that global obesity has doubled since 1980 (WHO, 2015). Coverage of the "obesity epidemic" is evident both in mainstream media (Leeds, 2010) and academic research (Mahmood & Arukumaran, 2013). Obesity has been described as a major public health concern due to the numerous health-related problems it is believed to cause. The UK National Health Service (NHS) links obesity to several life threatening conditions (e.g. type 2 diabetes, coronary heart diseases, stroke, some types of cancer, and depression (NHS, 2014)). Research linking obesity to a myriad of health problems is contested though. Romero-Corral et al. (2006) found that those classified as overweight or mildly obese based on BMI had better

DOI: 10.1057/9781137470461.0007

outcomes for cardiovascular and total mortality than those with a low BMI (<20). This has been called the "obesity paradox" and has generated considerable research, with some studies going as far as to suggest that "weight loss should not be the primary therapeutic goal for overweight and obese [heart failure] patients" (Clark, Fonarow, & Horwich, 2014, p.413). Although the public message about obesity and its dangers is clear, the reality is more nuanced.

There is now an onus on health professionals to encourage weight loss in overweight patients whatever their complaint. It is in the context of this uniform advice against an uncertain reality that the implications of the present research become clear. For those involved in feederism, their overweight body (or the body of their partner) is a key part of their sexual well-being. Their size is not the result of a lack of education about food or a poorly managed lifestyle, it is a choice that is likely to be a source of happiness rather than distress. Blachflower and Oswald (2004) demonstrated a significant relationship between sexual activity and happiness in a study of 16,000 Americans. Although more recent work by Loewenstein, Krishnamurti, Kopsic, and McDonald (2015) has disputed the direction of causation, there does seem to be good evidence that happiness and sex are linked on some level. If those involved in feederism are content with their choices, and it allows them to have fulfilling sexual relationships, then this should be seen as positive. A potential side effect of being overweight or obese is depression and low self-esteem. There should be greater awareness that for some individuals their size is a source of contentment that can have positive implications for their wider health.

Awareness of feederism amongst health professionals has not been measured but it is presumed to be low. Two participants in the current study said that there would be no help for them if they wanted to "leave" feederism because they felt medical professionals did not know about it. Other health professionals who were participants in the study described their dissonance over enjoying feederism yet being expected to promote messages of health. This is where greater awareness of the Health at Every Size (HAES, 2014) agenda could be effectively combined with traditional healthy living advice. Instead of focusing on weight, there could be a shift towards health, acknowledging that people can still have good cardiovascular health even when overweight or obese. In a randomized, controlled trial comparing two groups of sedentary overweight

DOI: 10.1057/9781137470461.0007

women taking part in an exercise programme, Hsu, Buckworth, Focht and Connell (2013) found that those who had received HAES orientation had significantly better adherence to physical activity goals and larger effect size changes in key motivational variables than the control group who only took part in the exercise programme. This demonstrates the potential health benefits of the HAES message to those who would not normally take part in physical activity. The HAES movement has inevitably faced some criticism, with Sainsbury and Hay (2014) arguing that there are limits to the concept and that it mostly relates to the overweight and mildly obese rather than those a BMI above 35.

Future research

Future research into feederism should attempt a quantitative study exploring the demographics and characteristics of feeders and feedees in greater detail. The advantage of this research would be a clearer understanding of the similarities that participants might share with one another, and it may help to further identify predictor variables relating to feederism. A quantitative approach would allow comparison with a general population group in a way that qualitative research cannot. It would also be interesting to undertake a prevalence study in order to understand how widespread feederism is.

There is also very little cross-cultural work on feederism. While some of the cultural differences in attitudes to fat women have been discussed in this text, specific differences in attitudes or participation in feederism are not known. Most of the participants in this research came from North America, with a small number coming from Europe. This geographical sampling is very similar to other research on feederism. The extent or practices of feederism in South America and Asia have not been explored by researchers even though there is considerable YouTube content on feederism with a Latin American theme as well as the Korean phenomenon of *mukbang* where individuals "perform" their eating through a webcam for a fee (Evans, 2015).

In the early stages of the current research, it was suggested by a reviewer that racial differences in feederism be explored. This was not possible in the current study because this information was not requested from participants. Further research could address this. It was similarly

DOI: 10.1057/9781137470461.0007

suggested that gay feederism should be explored. This was also suggested by participants in this study, and there is a lot of online content focused on gay gaining. Some female participants identified themselves as bisexual, but information on sexuality was not formally requested, so the present study cannot really offer any commentary on gay feederism. This could also be an area for further research.

There has been interesting work that has been developing in fat studies looking at using autoethnography as a way of exploring issues around embodiment, shame, identity management, and stigma through first-person accounts (Smailes, 2014). This development has been particularly focused around the idea of feminist knowledge creation strategies, such as documenting the lived experiences of larger women, who typically are not represented in academia. What could be useful is the same methodological strategy but used specifically to document deliberate weight gain strategies, perhaps with reference to literature developed in the sociology of the body (Schilling, 1993).

Future research could also assess the knowledge of feederism among health professionals, particularly those who are the first point of contact and who are often required to deliver healthy lifestyle messages (e.g. doctors and nurses who work in general practice in the UK). Carrying out survey-based research of this nature will identify whether training and awareness raising is needed. It is unrealistic to expect health professionals to promote being overweight, but knowing about feederism and the diversity of ways in which it is expressed may allow health professionals to tailor their approach to patients. In combination with the HAES agenda this would help feedees and mutual gainers stay healthy without stigmatizing them or expecting them to suppress their sexual desires.

References

Bancroft, J. & Marks, I. (1968). Electric Aversion Therapy of Sexual Deviations. *Proceedings of the Royal Society of Medicine, 61*, 796–799.

Beech, A. R., Craig, A. L., & Browne, K. D. (Eds.) (2009). *Assessment and Treatment of Sex Offenders*. Chichester: Wiley-Blackwell.

Blachflower, D. G. & Oswald, A. J. (2004). Money, Sex, and Happiness: An Empirical Study. *Scandinavian Journal of Economics, 10*, 393–415.

DOI: 10.1057/9781137470461.0007

Castelo-Branco, C., Huezo, M. L., & Lagarda, J. L. B. (2008). Definition and Diagnosis of Sexuality in the XXI Century. *Maturitas, 60*, 50–58.

Clark, A. L., Fonarow, G. C., & Horwich, T. B. (2014). Obesity and the Obesity Paradox in Heart Failure. *Progress in Cardiovascular Diseases, 56*, 409–414.

Evans, S. (2015). The Koreans Who Televise Themselves Eating Dinner. *BBC News*. Retrieved May 28, 2015, from http://www.bbc.co.uk/news/magazine-31130947.

HAES (2014). HAES UK. Retrieved May 28, 2015, from http://www.healthateverysize.org.uk/about.html.

Hsu, Y-T., Buckworth, J., Focht, B. C., & Connell, A. A. (2013). Feasibility of a Self-Determination Theory-Based Exercise Intervention Promoting Healthy at Every Size with Sedentary Overweight Women: Project CHANGE. *Psychology of Sport and Exercise, 14*, 283–292.

Långström, N., Babchishin, D. M., Fazel, S., Lichtenstein, P., & Frisell, T. (2015). Sexual Offending Runs in Families: A 37-Year Nationwide Study. *International Journal of Epidemiology, xx*, 1–8.

Leeds, T. (2010). Obesity: The Walking Financial Time Bomb. *BBC News*. Retrieved May 28, 2015, from http://news.bbc.co.uk/1/hi/health/8646677.stm.

Loewenstein, G., Krishnamurti, T., Kopsic, J., & McDonald, D. (2015). Does Increased Sexual Frequency Enhance Happiness? *Journal of Economic Behavior & Organization, 116*, 206–218.

Mahmood, T. & Arukumaran, S. (Eds.) (2013). *Obesity*. London: Elsevier.

NHS (2014). Obesity. Retrieved May 28, 2015, from http://www.nhs.uk/Conditions/Obesity/Pages/Introduction.aspx.

Oliver, J. E. (2006). *Fat Politics: The Real Story behind America's Obesity Epidemic*. New York: Oxford University Press.

Pettinger, A. (1993). Why Fetish? *New Formations, 19*, 88–93.

Prohaska, A. (2013). Feederism: Transgressive Behavior or Same Old Patriarchal Sex? *International Journal of Social Science Studies, 1*, 104–112.

Romero-Corral, A., Montori, V. M., Somers, V. K., Korinek, J., Thomas, R. J., Allison, T. G., Mookadam, F., & Lopez-Jimenez, F. (2006). Association of Bodyweight with Total Mortality and with Cardiovascular Events in Coronary Artery Disease: A Systematic Review of Cohort Studies. *The Lancet, 368*, 666–678.

DOI: 10.1057/9781137470461.0007

Sainsbury, A. & Hay, P. (2014). Call for an Urgent Rethink of the "Health at Every Size" Concept. *Journal of Eating Disorders*, 2, 8.

Shilling, C. (1993). *The Body and Social Theory*. London: Sage.

Smailes, S. (2014). Negotiating and Navigating My Fat Body – Feminist Autoethnographic Encounters. *Athenea Digital. Revista de pensamiento e investigación social*, *14*, 49.

WHO (2015). Obesity and Overweight. *World Health Organization*. Retrieved May 28, 2015, from http://www.who.int/mediacentre/factsheets/fs311/en/.

Willy Wonka & the Chocolate Factory [Motion picture]. (1971). USA: Paramount.

Wilson, S. & MacLean, R. (2011). *Research Methods and Data Analysis for Psychology*. New York: McGraw-Hill.

DOI: 10.1057/9781137470461.0007

Index

900 Club, 3

addiction
  brain disease model of (BDMA), 14–16
  feederism, 14
  food, 14–15
  sex, 14, 16
agency, 81, 82–4
authenticity, 75–6, 76–7
autoerotic feeding, 10, 24–5, 27, 47–8, 61, 67, 71–2, 75

BDMA (brain disease model of addiction), 14–16
BDSM, 50, 60, 66, 68
Bestard, A., 17–20, 24, 26, 29, 34
BMI (Body Mass Index), 9–10, 68, 94–6
body habitus, 23, 26
Body Panopticon, 20
body project, 20, 27, 29, 33

cartoons, fat intrigue, 45–6
Clips4Sale, 61, 71, 72, 83
commercial autoeroticism, 71–2
couples
  fetish/sexuality, 79–80
  interviews of, 76–80
  narratives, 77–8
culture of slenderness, 22, 29–30, 78

Dimensions (magazine) website, 3, 22, 43, 85, 87
dominant gainer, 58
domination, 3–4, 31, 52, 61, 67, 70, 82–3, 93

extremefeeding.com, 4–5, 41, 53

family
  conflict, 7, 73–4, 91
  humiliation, 61–2
  life, 18, 72
  secrecy, 49–50, 70
  tainted, 90–1
Fantasy Feeder, 3, 13–14, 26, 49, 72, 75
fat
  co-constructed, 86–7
  feminist studies, 30–1
  representation, 44–6
  stigmatization and, 18–19
"Fat Girls and Feeders" (documentary), 5–6, 56
Fat is a Feminist Issue (Susie Orbach), 30–1
Feabie.com, 56
feedee, labelling, 46–9
feederism
  dominant gainer, 58
  early experiences, 54, 63, 65, 72
  extreme, 50–1, 55, 59–60, 64, 66, 68, 70
  future research, 96–7

DOI: 10.1057/9781137470461.0008

feederism – *continued*
humiliation, 60–2
immobility, 4–5, 9, 22, 25, 30, 50–1, 55, 59–61, 64, 66, 68, 70, 81, 83–4, 87
importance of food, 58–9
intersections of sex and fat, 27–8
labelling, 46–9
lifestyle, 2, 3, 17, 19, 23, 28, 30, 56, 70
limitations of health frame, 71
mainstream representations of, 3–7
meaning of, 54, 63, 65, 67, 69
online presence, 59
practical applications, 94–6
promoting alternative views, 55–6, 57
psychological research, 7–16
public narrative, 51–2
role fluidity, 71
sociological research, 16–24
sociological studies of, 24–33
terminology, 2–3
theoretical contribution, 90–2
treatments, 90–1
"Feed" (film), 6–7
feeding identity, 34
femininity, 20–1, 30–1, 55
feminist studies
fat, 30–1
feederism, 33
fetish, 3–7, 19, 29–31, 46–52, 55, 61, 68, 79–80, 91
food
addiction, 14–16
importance of, 58–9
meaning of, 64, 65–6
as means to an end, 72–3
force-feeding, 4, 9, 11–12, 26, 28, 50–1, 55, 64, 66, 68, 81, 83, 86
Foucault, M., 19–20, 22–3, 25, 28
funnel-feeding, 42, 50, 60–1, 64, 66, 68, 70, 73, 83

habitus, 23
Health at Every Size agenda, 22, 48, 69, 95, 96, 97
health professionals, feederism awareness, 95, 97
hedonism, 73–4
Horngry (online magazine), 4, 41, 55–6, 57
humiliation, 60–2

immobility, 4–5, 9, 22, 25, 30, 50–1, 55, 59–61, 64, 66, 68, 70, 81, 83–4, 87
interviews
limitations for recruitment, 92–3
participants, 43
public narrative, 51–2
schedule, 42–3
semi-structured, 41–2, 52–81
stories, 43
written responses, 43–52
see also semi-structured interviews
interviews, themes of
agency, 81, 82–4
dominant gainer, 58
early experiences, 63, 67, 69, 72, 73, 75
early life and humiliation, 60–2
extreme, 50–1, 55, 59–60, 64, 66, 68, 70
family conflict, 73–4
fat representations, 44–6
food, importance of, 58–9, 64, 65–6
food, means to an end, 72–3
hedonism, 73–4
internet exchange, 75–6
placing oneself, 74–5
labelling, 46–9, 56, 58
loss of control, 62
online presence, 59
pillows, 44
promoting alternative views, 55–6, 57
secrecy, 49–50, 64, 66, 68, 70

labelling, feederism, 9, 46–9, 56, 58
leblouh tradition, 8

masculinity, 21, 30, 58–9, 86
masturbation, 67, 69, 92

DOI: 10.1057/9781137470461.0008

NAAFA (National Association to Advance Fat Acceptance), 8, 25
narratives, *see* interviews; stories
NHS (National Health Service), 6, 94

obesity, 8, 18, 21, 22, 52, 69, 94–5
obesity epidemic, 94
obesity paradox, 95
online presence
  dark side of, 75–6
  feederism, 59

panopticon, 19–20
paraphilia, feederism as, 2, 8–10, 41, 79, 91
participants
  limitations for recruitment, 92–3
  see also interviews, themes of; semi-structured interviews
patriarchal dynamics, 28, 41, 60
patriarchal power, 24, 41
patriarchal sex, 25, 31, 33, 60
patriarchy, 16, 33, 82
"Pigs is Pigs" cartoon, 11–12, 67, 78, 91
power, 13, 19, 22, 24, 25–6, 28–9, 34, 41, 58–9, 74, 82, 84
Prohaska, A., 4, 20, 25–7, 31, 33, 53, 60
public narrative, feederism, 51–2

research, future, 96–7

sadomasochism, 4, 9–10, 90
secrecy, feederism, 49–50, 64, 66, 68, 70
semi-structured interviews, 41–2
  agency, 81, 82–4
  Ashley, 71–3
  Benny, 66–8
  Blossom, 74–6
  couples, 76–80
  Dorothy and Dwight, 79–80
  Gabriela, 56, 58–60
  Gavin, 69–70
  Gemma, 65–6
  Grayson, 60–2
  James, 73–4
  Reginald and Wendy, 79–80
  Ruben, 53–6
  Saskia, 63–4
  Virginia and Terrance, 76–9
  see also interviews, themes of
sex addiction, 14, 16
sexual arousal, food as, 7, 9, 13
sexuality
  couples, 79–80
  deviant, 17, 20, 22–3, 24, 30, 79, 90
  framing of, 23–4, 26
  human, 91–2
  intersections of sex and fat, 27–8
slenderness, culture of, 22, 29–30, 78
spoiled identity, 18
stories, 43
  co-constructed fat, 86–7
  fattest in the world, 87
  men gaining: female feeding, 84–6
  weight, 84
  see also interviews, themes of
symbolic interactionism, 17–18

Terry, Lesley, 7–10, 13–14, 20
tube-feeding, 4, 42, 50, 60–1, 64, 66, 68, 70, 73, 83

weight stories, 84
  co-constructed fat, 86–7
  men gaining: female feeding, 84–6
  see also interviews
Willy Wonka and the Chocolate Factory (movie), 45, 63, 91

DOI: 10.1057/9781137470461.0008

www.ingramcontent.com/pod-product-compliance
Lightning Source LLC
Chambersburg PA
CBHW060741120826
49620CB00036B/14
* 9 7 8 1 1 3 7 4 7 0 4 5 4 *